Neurological Therapeutics

Neurological Therapeutics

D L W Davidson BSc, MB, ChB, FRCP Ed
*Consultant Neurologist, Dundee Royal Infirmary and
Ninewells Hospital, Dundee; Honorary Senior Lecturer
in Neurology, Dundee University*

J A R Lenman MB, ChB, FRCP Ed, FRSE
*Reader in Neurology, Dundee University; Honorary
Consultant Neurologist, Dundee Royal Infirmary and
Ninewells Hospital, Dundee*

PITMAN MEDICAL

First published 1981

Catalogue Number 21 2204 81

Pitman Medical Limited
39 Parker Street, London WC2B 5PB

Associated Companies
Pitman Publishing Pty Ltd, Melbourne
Pitman Publishing New Zealand Ltd, Wellington

© D L W Davidson and J A R Lenman, 1981

British Library Cataloguing in Publication Data

Davidson, D. L. W.
   Neurological therapeutics.
   1. Neurology
   I. Title   II. Lenman, J. A. R.
   616.8   RC346

ISBN: 0-272-79616-6

Set in 11/12 pt IBM Journal by
Freeman Graphic, Tonbridge
Printed and bound in Great Britain
at The Pitman Press, Bath

Contents

Preface

The aim of this book is to draw together views on the therapy of neurological disorders to provide a useful exposition of current treatment suitable for neurologists in training, physicians in hospital and general practitioners. It is hoped that it will be helpful to students and also to practitioners in other fields who from time to time may be faced with a neurological problem.

Although many neurological disorders remain resistant to specific therapy there have been important advances particularly in respect of conditions such as infections, epilepsy, and disorders of movement where effective drug treatment has become available and developments in technique have widened the scope of surgery. Moreover in conditions which remain intractable much can be done to alleviate the situation of the patient by appropriate management. In the present account the use of drugs, the indications for surgery, and the role of intensive care and rehabilitation are discussed. Evidence is presented in the discussion of controversial topics and selected references are provided at the end of each chapter. Some knowledge of clinical neurology is assumed and therefore reference is made to clinical features, pathophysiological mechanisms, and investigations only when these are important in the application of therapy. The genetics of inherited disorders and the natural history of progressive disorders are outlined because these are important in the management of patients. No detailed account of paediatric or psychiatric topics is included except where these seem relevant to conditions presenting in the general neurological clinic.

It is a pleasure to acknowledge the help which we have received from many sources. In particular we should like to thank Dr Mary Kerr for her helpful comments on the treatment of infections, and Mrs Norma Spain and Miss Karile Janavicius for typing the manuscript. We are grateful to authors and publishers who have generously granted permission to reproduce illustrations. In each case the source is acknowledged in the caption. Finally, we should like to thank Mr Stephen Neal, Mr Graham Smith and the staff of Pitman Medical for their help and co-operation.

Dundee
June 1980

D.L.W.D.
J.A.R.L.

CHAPTER ONE

General Principles of Therapy

Although many chronic disorders of the nervous system are as yet without any specific cure, or indeed have no specific therapy which will modify the course of the disease, there are many patients who have illnesses which are not in the strict sense curable but who yet require considerable medical assistance over the years if they are to cope with the problems of the disease. Nevertheless, specific drug therapy is now available in the treatment of a substantial number of disorders and others are amenable to surgical treatment. Although the physician is not concerned with the details of operative procedure, in a number of conditions, both medical and surgical measures may be indicated according to the clinical situation and it is important to appreciate the circumstances in which surgical intervention may be indicated. In addition to pharmacological and surgical therapy the management of neurological disorders may depend upon the application of a variety of special techniques such as, for example, those of physiotherapy, speech therapy, psychotherapy, and occupational therapy. Moreover in the management of an illness, although little may appear to be possible to modify the course of the disease, it is still necessary to have an accurate diagnosis if one is to explain the prognosis to the patient or the patient's relatives so that appropriate adaptations and adjustments can be made. Many disorders have a genetic basis and where this is the case accurate knowledge not only of the natural history of the disease but of the genetic mechanisms governing its inheritance is necessary if appropriate advice and counselling are to be given to the patient or to the patient's close relatives.

DRUG THERAPY

Drugs which are effective in neurological disease include analgesics for the relief of pain, sedatives for the control of mood and behaviour, anticonvulsants, drugs which relieve muscle spasm, antibiotics, and drugs which modify neurotransmission both in the brain and in the peripheral nervous system. Drugs which are beneficial in therapeutic doses may have adverse effects if the dose is excessive, whereas others may give rise to harmful effects if the patient is idiosyncratic or hypersensitive. Some drugs which are normally beneficial will harm the fetus if taken by the mother during the first 6 weeks of pregnancy. Some drugs can be given effectively along with other forms of medication but with many combinations of drugs interactions occur which may affect the efficacy of one or both forms of medication. Drugs vary greatly in their rate of absorption, in the duration of time in which they persist in the body, and in their distribution throughout the body fluids; with some drugs it is particularly important to measure their concentration in the blood if effective therapy is to be maintained. In later sections of this book the clinical pharmacology of particular drugs will be considered, where relevant, in connection with the particular disorders for which they are indicated.

PHARMACODYNAMICS

In studying the therapeutic actions of a drug it is important to be able to measure the therapeutic effect in terms of the dose required to achieve that effect. The effect may be a clinical one such as, for example, the effect of a hypnotic in producing sleep or a biochemical effect such as the effect of a chelating agent in ridding the body of a foreign substance. With a particular drug the pharmacodynamics can be expressed in terms of a dose—response curve.

PHARMACOKINETICS

The pharmacokinetics of a drug refers to the rate at which it is absorbed, how it is distributed throughout the body, how it is metabolised and finally excreted. If the action of a drug depends on its concentration in the plasma it is important that its rate of absorption should be sufficient to obtain an adequate concentration. The distribution of the drug throughout the different compartments of the body fluids is important in terms of its therapeutic action. Thus some drugs if taken by mouth become uniformly distributed throughout the body fluids, whereas others maintain a differential concentration between the different compartments. Of particular importance in the nervous system is the ease with which substances pass through the blood—brain barrier. Thus certain antibiotics such as penicillin will not readily enter the nervous system if given by intramuscular injection. Dopamine if taken by mouth does not pass from the blood stream into the brain but its precursor levodopa will do so and break down there to give rise to pharmacologically active dopamine. Some drugs are excreted unchanged but many are metabolised, for example, in the liver to be converted into pharmacologically inactive substances prior to excretion. Others break down into substances which have a different but nevertheless important pharmacological action such as, for example, phenobarbitone which is formed when primidone is broken down in the liver. If liver function is impaired, therapeutic concentrations of a drug may become toxic. With some drugs the metabolic rate may have a considerable effect on the therapeutic action. Thus, for example, with phenytoin the enzymes which metabolise it may reach a point where they become saturated and at this stage a small increase in the amount of phenytoin in the body may lead to the development of high and possibly toxic blood levels. The excretion of drugs is generally through the kidneys and again it is important to recognise that in renal failure high and possibly toxic doses of a drug may build up through inadequate excretion. The rate of absorption, metabolism, and excretion of a drug determine both the rate at which an effective plasma concentration is reached and the length of time the drug will persist in the body. This length of time is expressed as the plasma half-life of a drug which is the time taken for the concentration to fall by 50 per cent, and is a useful guide to how frequently the drug must be administered to be effective. Thus phenytoin has a long half-life and a period of some days may be necessary before the drug reaches an effective plasma level. Once this level is reached it may be maintained by giving the drug in single or twice-daily doses. On the other hand, carbamazepine has a short half-life, its clinical effect is rapidly achieved, but it must be given in frequent divided doses if effective blood concentrations are to be maintained.

PHARMACOGENETICS

Different individuals may respond to drugs in different ways. This is not necessarily genetically determined. Thus, for example, a patient with renal failure may develop signs of neuropathy after taking nitrofurantoin; and young babies and the very old may be intolerant of morphine. Other differences, however, are genetically determined. Thus, for example, the drug isoniazid is inactivated by acetylation and some people inactivate it rapidly whereas others inactivate it slowly. Slow inactivators have blood levels which remain high for considerably longer than rapid inactivators who take the same dose. Since isoniazid inhibits microsomal hydroxylation of phenytoin (Kutt *et al.*, 1968) slow acetylators may be more likely to develop phenytoin toxicity if they take both drugs. It would appear that slow inactivators are more likely to develop toxic symptoms than are rapid inactivators — symptoms such as, for example, peripheral neuropathy — and it is known that the gene carried by slow inactivators is an autosomal recessive. Malignant hyperpyrexia, on the other hand, in which susceptible patients develop hyperthermia during anaesthesia with halothane and succinylcholine, is inherited as an autosomal dominant.

DRUG INTERACTIONS

Drug interactions can occur before administration of the drug. This is particularly liable to be a problem if drugs are administered by intravenous infusion, when interactions may give rise to precipitation. Thus drugs such as barbiturates, heparin, phenothiazines, phenytoin, and vitamin B complex should not be mixed with any other drugs in solution. Some drugs may interfere with the absorption of others in the gastrointestinal tract. In the blood stream drugs may compete for protein-binding sites. An important example is the competition which occurs with phenylbutazone and warfarin since phenylbutazone can displace warfarin from its binding site and give rise to haemorrhage. Certain drugs will activate the microsomal hepatic enzymes which are concerned with drug inactivation. Barbiturates are very effective enzyme inducers and may increase the rate of metabolism of other drugs such as warfarin or phenytoin. Both phenobarbitone and phenytoin by this means may alter the activity of oral contraceptives, so that if a patient is taking an oral contraceptive along with anticonvulsant therapy the oral contraceptive, to be fully effective, should be one containing more than the usual amounts of both oestrogen and progesterone. Drugs may also potentiate the activity of other drugs by inhibiting drug-metabolising enzymes. Thus the monoamine oxidase inhibitors may delay the metabolism of sympathomimetic amines and enhance the effect of catecholamines released by drugs such as ephedrine. They may also prevent the destruction of tyramine in foods such as cheese, so that food containing tyramine can give rise to a hypertensive crisis. Drugs can also interfere with each other by competing for the receptor on which they act; thus chlorpromazine may interfere with the action of levodopa, and nalorphine will reverse morphine narcosis by competing with the receptor site of the morphine. Other drugs antagonise each other at the final site of operation in a different manner; thus certain hypotensive drugs such as guanethidine block adrenergic transmission by promoting the uptake of catecholamines. This action, however, may be inhibited by chlorpromazine and the tricyclic antidepressants which may therefore reverse the effect on hypertension of these drugs.

TERATOGENICITY

A number of drugs have been found to have an adverse effect on the fetus if taken by a pregnant woman during the first trimester of pregnancy. Examples of such drugs are thalidomide and warfarin, but the difficulty of testing drugs to rule out a possible teratogenic effect means that it is unwise to administer any drug which has newly been introduced to women of child-bearing age who may become pregnant. Studies carried out on women with epilepsy have shown that those who have epilepsy under treatment with anticonvulsants, apparently particularly with phenytoin, have a slightly greater risk of having a child with a congenital abnormality, particularly hair lip or cleft palate. Against this risk, however, must be balanced the dangers to the mother and fetus if the mother should have seizures in the absence of adequate therapy. The critical period for teratogenic effects on the nervous system is between the 15th and 25th days of gestation. After the period of organogenesis drugs may affect growth and function of normally formed tissues and organs. Thus long-acting sulphonamides may displace bilirubin from its binding sites and give rise to jaundice and kernicterus.

SURGICAL TREATMENT

In a book concerned with therapeutics no detailed consideration can be given to the technical aspects of surgical treatment, and for detailed accounts of the indications for surgery in the management of neurological disorders the reader is referred to books on surgical neurology. In many areas of neurology, however, both medical treatment and neurosurgery are essential in the management of the patient and for this reason some discussion is given to the indications for appropriate surgical treatment in the relevant clinical sections.

The recognition of surgically treatable conditions is an important part of the investigation and management of patients who present with neurological symptoms, and judgement is frequently called for in deciding how far it is appropriate to advise a patient to submit to invasive and possibly hazardous investigations in order to establish a definitive diagnosis. The criterion in this situation must always be the benefit which will ultimately accrue to the patient, and this needs to be balanced against the possible hazards of investigation and operation. Fortunately the development of new non-invasive methods of investigation such as computerised axial tomography has made the situation less difficult, at least in respect of intracranial disease.

PHYSIOTHERAPY

The methods of physiotherapy are essential in the treatment of patients with motor impairment. Thus a patient with an acute paralytic lesion due, for example, to a stroke requires passive movements of the paralysed limb from the outset of paralysis to prevent the development of stiffness and contractures. As power returns the patient must be taught to carry out active movements and the skills of the physiotherapist are necessary if the patient is to be mobilised and taught to walk independently. In patients with paraplegia or severe spasticity physiotherapy, again largely in the form of passive movements, is necessary to overcome muscle spasm. The patient confined to bed, or with severe paralysis, may also require assistance in coughing and in carrying out breathing exercises and in proper positioning of the chest; this is of particular importance in patients who require assisted ventilation. In patients with progressive disorders of the nervous system such as Parkinson's disease, Friedreich's ataxia or multiple sclerosis, periodic courses of physiotherapy may be of value hopefully to restore function where this has been lost, but often also to enable patients to learn (by new techniques of walking or the use of appliances such as tripods and other forms of walking aid) to adapt to their disability so they can remain mobile if their condition changes. With rapidly progressive conditions such as motor neurone disease physiotherapy must be used with caution, as failure to carry out prescribed exercises may merely draw the patient's attention to the advance of the disease. In the rehabilitation of patients following a neurosurgical operation physiotherapy again may be essential in enabling the patient to walk and become mobile. In cervical spondylosis and lumbar disc lesions active shoulder girdle exercises and back extension exercises may assist in the patient's recovery and mobilisation and in peripheral nerve lesions active exercises in association with the provision of appropriate splints may be helpful in maintaining function until recovery has taken place. The use of electrotherapy remains somewhat controversial. There is no doubt that the application of heat in the form of diathermy or infrared radiation will bring comfort to patients with inflammatory lesions. The value of electrical stimulation of paralysed muscles in promoting recovery is less certain, although there seems no doubt that it is effective in preventing muscle wasting (*see* Chapter 12). Other forms of physical therapy which are

important, but are more the province of the physical medicine physician, include traction and manipulation which judiciously applied may
have a place in the management of cervical and lumbar spondylosis.
Biofeedback, in which the patient learns to modify muscle activity in
response to signals from his own electromyogram (EMG), is a relatively
new technique which may be useful in the treatment of spasticity and
disorders of motor control (Basmajian, 1979).

SPEECH THERAPY

Although much of the work of a speech therapist is devoted to the careful education of children whose ability to communicate is handicapped
by deafness or by cerebral palsy, speech therapy also has an important
place in the management of adults who have become dysphasic as a
result of neurological disease — particularly in cerebrovascular episodes.
Much here depends upon the ability of the patient to co-operate and on
how far there is a natural tendency for recovery. Where recovery of
verbal communication is not possible the speech therapist can contribute greatly by teaching the patient methods of non-verbal communication.

OCCUPATIONAL THERAPY

Occupational therapy is also of value in the management of patients
with a chronic neurological disability. These patients can be taught
activities such as, for example, those requiring the use of fine movements which will enable the patient to develop useful function as
recovery takes place. Once a moderate degree of recovery has taken
place the occupational therapist will help the patient to adapt to
activities in the home, particularly in the kitchen, and at work. Where
the patient has severe continuing disability the occupational therapist
will also assess the requirements of the patient in terms of adaptations
to the home, wheelchairs and, if necessary, electronic aids such as the
possum (patient operated selector mechanism) apparatus.

THE UNCONSCIOUS PATIENT

Two situations where the demands on neurological nursing are particularly heavy are in the care of the paraplegic patient and in the management of the patient who is unconscious. Care of paraplegia is dealt with
in Chapter 15. In the management of the unconscious patient it is
essential at the outset to establish an adequate airway. The patient

should be turned on his side to prevent the tongue falling back, and suction should be applied to remove secretions from the mouth and pharynx and respiratory passages. In the early stages the gastric contents should be aspirated with an intranasal tube and if unconsciousness is at all prolonged tracheal intubation is advisable; if this has to be continued for more than 7 days then a tracheostomy may be advisable. Physiotherapy is essential to remove secretions and the patient must be turned frequently to avoid the development of pressure sores. It may be advisable to give an antibiotic to prevent chest infection and regular examination of the urine must be carried out — both to ascertain that there is an adequate urinary output and to detect infection. Intravenous fluid may be necessary to maintain adequate hydration and the serum electrolytes must be estimated every day. Adequate food intake and fluid intake can usually be maintained through a nasogastric tube.

The medical management of the unconscious patient has been reviewed in detail by Plum and Posner (1972). A very full examination is required both in order to determine the cause of the unconscious state and to monitor the patient so that appropriate management decisions can be made and prognosis can be assessed. The history and presentation may distinguish between major causes of unconsciousness such as head injury, brain tumour, cerebral haemorrhage or infarct or status epilepticus but laboratory screening will be necessary to identify infective or metabolic causes such as, for example, meningitis, drug intoxication, uraemia or diabetes. X-rays of skull, EEG, isotope scanning, CAT scanning and sometimes angiography may be indicated to define an intracranial lesion such as a tumour, blood clot or aneurysm. Lumbar puncture is necessary if there is any possibility of intracranial infection or abscess but great caution must be exercised if there is papilloedema or other evidence of raised intracranial pressure in view of the risk of precipitating tentorial or foraminal impaction.

Accurate assessment and documentation of the level of consciousness initially and at regular intervals is of paramount importance in monitoring the patient's condition. The level of consciousness may be defined as *coma* if the patient is unable to respond to painful stimuli, or as *stupor* if he responds to vigorous stimulation. In prolonged coma the patient may pass into a state of non-cognitive wakefulness or *vegetative state* (Jennett and Plum, 1972) in which the eyes are open and primitive responses occur. In lighter states of unconsciousness the patient will obey simple commands, respond to questions and be orientated for time and place but drowsy. If he is disorientated the condition is known as *confusion*, or as *delirium* if he is also disturbed and perhaps hallucinated. *Coma* must be distinguished from *akinetic mutism*, where

OBSERVATION CHART FOR COMA

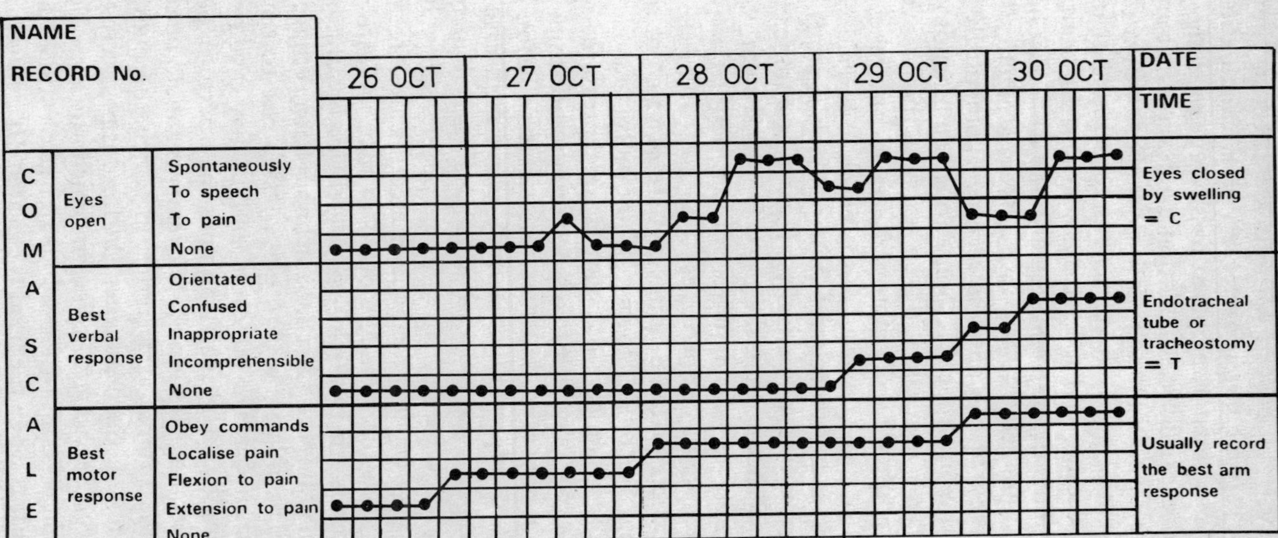

Figure 1.1 Nursing chart to record level of coma (see text). Only five motor responses are included in this simplified scale. Reproduced by kind permission of G Teasdale, W B Jennett and the Editor of the *Nursing Times*

the patient lies still and silent but may follow movements with his eyes and which may be associated with disease affecting the diencephalon, and from *psychogenic unresponsiveness* where the patient appears unconscious but may resist attempts at passive eye-opening, and where the EEG is normal and caloric stimulation evokes a quick and a slow component. In the de-efferentated state or *locked-in syndrome*, due to a lesion in the ventral pons, the patient is conscious but unable to communicate on account of total paralysis except for ventral eye movements and blinking. In this condition also the EEG may be normal.

Teasdale and Jennett (1974) have devised a practical coma scale in which a hierarchy of responses is recorded numerically in three components, viz., the best motor response (obey commands — localise pain — flexion to pain — extension to pain — none), the best verbal response (orientated — confused — inappropriate — incomprehensible — none) and eye opening (spontaneously — to speech — to pain — none). These parameters are readily incorporated in a nurse's chart (*see* Figure 1.1) and can also be ranked numerically by giving a number higher by one for each response better than the next. In this system, which has been applied specifically to head injuries, *coma* is defined as failure to obey commands, utter words or open eyes.

Particular aspects of the examination are of value in the assessment and monitoring of coma. Slowing of the pulse and elevation of the blood pressure may indicate rising intracranial pressure, as may slowing of the respirations. Cheyne—Stokes or periodic breathing may occur in deep coma from any cause but may also signify a lesion in the diencephalon. Sustained hyperventilation may occur in disease affecting the midbrain or the pons, and in metabolic acidosis as in diabetes or uraemia. Irregular or ataxic breathing in which respirations vary both in depth and frequency may occur if the pons or medulla are affected. Failure to evoke a blink by a threatening movement may indicate a field defect and ophthalmoscopy may disclose papilloedema or subhyaloid haemorrhages which may be seen after subarachnoid haemorrhage. A unilateral dilated pupil may indicate a IIIrd nerve lesion due to tentorial herniation and midbrain damage or severe anoxia may give rise to bilateral fixed dilated pupils. Small reactive pupils may occur in pontine lesions or in opiate poisoning. Reflex eye movements should be recorded, viz., the *oculocephalic* (*doll's head*) reflex in which the eyes move in the opposite direction to the head when the head is passively turned to one side, and the *oculovestibular reflex* in which the eyes deviate to the irrigated side when 20 ml of ice-cold water are instilled into the external auditory meatus when the head is elevated 30° above the horizontal. In this test the tympanic membrane must first be visualised to confirm that it is intact. Absence of either of these reflexes may indicate a lesion in the pons or midbrain but either may be lost in poisoning by sedative drugs such as barbiturates.

The outcome of coma may vary between complete recovery and a continued vegetative state or death, with intermediate stages with varying degrees of disability and dependency. The prognosis may be assessed both in respect of the underlying disease and the clinical condition of the patient. Criteria for determining prognosis in coma resulting from head injury have been reviewed by Jennett *et al.* (1978) and from medical causes by Caronna *et al.* (1978). In coma due to epilepsy or to intoxication with barbiturates or alcohol many patients can be expected to recover but persistent coma following cerebral haemorrhage, acute hepatic failure, purulent meningitis or cardiac arrest carries a high mortality. In general the longer the duration of coma the poorer the outcome, and relatively few will recover when coma has been present for more than a week. Signs such as eye-opening with blinking and sustained regular respiration are favourable signs but fixed pupils, absent corneal, oculocephalic and oculovestibular reflexes or appropriate motor responses are all consistent with a poor outlook unless there is evidence also of drug intoxication. Reliable prediction of outcome, however, in the early stages remains difficult and great caution must be exercised in reaching any therapeutic decision which is based on an estimation of prognosis.

ARTIFICIAL VENTILATION

Where there is paralysis of the respiratory or bulbar muscles then artificial ventilation may be necessary. This may arise in conditions such as poliomyelitis, post-infective polyneuritis, transverse myelitis, polymyositis, myasthenia gravis and sometimes in severe status epilepticus or in multiple sclerosis if the bulbar muscles are affected. Where a person's respiration is precarious it is advisable to start artificial ventilation early rather than late, and blood gas analysis may be helpful in assessing when this is necessary. Clinical assessment of a patient's respiratory function can be carried out by recording the patient's peak flow expiratory capacity, forced expiratory volume or vital capacity at regular intervals. It is generally not advisable to start artificial ventilation unless the patient's illness allows some prospect of recovery and it is generally not advisable to start it in the terminally ill. In conditions where the outcome is in doubt, as in the unconscious patient after a severe head injury, then exceedingly difficult problems in management may arise. Generally speaking patients on artificial ventilation should be treated in an intensive care unit and the method now employed is that of intermittent positive pressure respiration which unlike the tank respirator is able to cope with bulbar paralysis as well as paralysis of the respiratory muscles. The patient receiving artificial ventilation requires all the facilities in terms of intensive nursing care and physiotherapy which are given to the paralysed and comatose patient.

BRAIN DEATH

If a patient is comatose, as a result of severe brain damage, and maintained on a ventilator the situation may arise that the brain ceases to function but the circulation continues while respiration is maintained artificially. In this situation of brain death cardiovascular function will generally cease within a matter of days and the brain at autopsy will show widespread autolysis — the 'respirator brain'. This condition is distinct from that of coma, or a vegetative state, which may be irreversible, but where life may continue sometimes for long periods. Its recognition is important because on the one hand it may make it possible to avoid the needless continuation of intensive care, and on the other hand the recognition of brain death before cardiac arrest may enable organs of good quality to be obtained for transplant.

The terminology used in considering brain death has been reviewed by Korein (1978). The term *brain death* may be taken to include destruction of the neuronal contents of the cranial cavity including the cerebral hemispheres, the deep midline structures, the brainstem and cerebellum. The term *cerebral death* is sometimes used synonymously but may be used also to cover the uncommon situation where the cerebral hemispheres alone are involved with preservation of the brainstem. Likewise there may exist a situation of *brainstem death* in which brainstem function is absent but there may be some evidence of electroencephalographic activity or cerebral circulation. The term *neocortical death* or *apallic syndrome* has been used to describe states where there is widespread loss of cortical neurones in each hemisphere with preservation of the deep nuclei and brainstem. This may be associated with a wide variety of clinical states such as prolonged and sometimes irreversible coma and vegetative states.

The diagnosis of brain death depends firstly on establishing that the brain has been severely damaged by a condition which may be fatal, such as head injury, cardiac arrest or stroke, and is not the result of drug intoxication, hypothermia or metabolic disturbance. Moreover all reasonable means must have been adopted to treat the patient including maintenance of respiration on a ventilator. Codes of practice which have been adopted to assist in the diagnosis of brain death include the Harvard criteria (Beecher, 1968) and the 1976 statement of the Conference of Medical Royal Colleges of Great Britain and their Faculties. Recent reviews include those of Glaser (1978) and Posner (1978).

The statement of the Conference of Medical Royal Colleges, to which the reader is referred, lists as three prerequisites that the patient must be deeply comatose, is maintained on a ventilator because spontaneous respiration has ceased or is inadequate, and has been shown to have irremediable brain damage due to a disorder which can lead to brain death. Depressant drugs, muscular relaxants, endocrine or metabolic disturbance and hypothermia must have been excluded as possible causes. Furthermore it must be shown that brainstem reflexes are absent as evidenced by non-reactive pupils; absent corneal, vestibulo-ocular and gag reflexes; and absence of any motor response within the cranial nerve distribution to sensory stimulation. In addition there must be no respiratory movements when the patient is disconnected from the ventilator long enough to ensure that the arterial CO_2 concentration rises above the threshold for respiratory stimulation. This is best undertaken using blood gas analysis but if this is not possible the patient should be given pure oxygen for 10 min followed by 5 per cent CO_2 in oxygen for 5 min through the respirator, which is then disconnected for 10 min while oxygen is delivered at 6 l/min by catheter into the trachea. In contrast to brainstem reflexes spinal reflexes such as the tendon jerks may persist in brain-dead patients.

In general it is advisable to repeat the tests to rule out observer error after an interval of 12–24 h. A valuable confirmatory sign is the demonstration of an isoelectric EEG on at least two occasions. The EEG examination must be carried out with meticulous care to avoid contamination by artefact and it is recommended that the strict criteria outlined by the International Federation of Societies for EEG and Clinical Neurophysiology (1974) be followed. It must be recognised, moreover, that a flat EEG may be present for as long as 48 h in severe drug intoxication. Angiographic demonstration of an absent cerebral circulation may provide definitive confirmation of brain death but is not generally necessary if strict clinical criteria are observed.

There are many pitfalls in the diagnosis of brain death and it is advisable that the decision to withdraw artificial support after the criteria have been fulfilled should be made by two doctors in consultation. The statement of the Conference of Medical Royal Colleges specifies that one of these should be the consultant in charge of the case, or his deputy, who must have been registered for at least 5 years. If organ transplantation is contemplated neither physician should be a member of the transplant team.

GENETIC COUNSELLING

A number of neurological disorders show a tendency to occur in families, and where this is the case patients or their close relatives may require advice concerning the risk of their having affected children. The main importance of this is in the prevention of disease but it is also relevant to treatment since a number of inborn errors of metabolism can be given effective treatment if recognised sufficiently early. Two such examples are phenylketonuria and Wilson's disease. Effective genetic counselling involves both accurate diagnosis and understanding of the mode of inheritance. A number of common conditions such as epilepsy have what is called a multifactorial inheritance, which depends usually on the effect of more than one gene, the expression of which may also be influenced by environmental factors. Where this is so the incidence in affected relatives can only be determined empirically. It must be borne in mind, when advising patients with a disease which is inherited on a multifactorial basis, that the incidence is considerably higher among close relatives of the patient than in the general population. Thus with epilepsy the overall incidence is of the order of 0.5 per cent but may be as high as 5 per cent of relatives of an affected patient. Where the illness is inherited through a single gene (unifactorial) it may be possible to give a precise estimate of the probability of an individual being a carrier, or of the patient having affected children. The posterior or relative probability of an individual having inherited a condition or being a carrier may be calculated according to Bayes' theorem in which the relative probability is the joint probability of being affected (or being a carrier) divided by the joint probability of not being affected plus the joint probability of being affected. The joint probability is the product of the prior and conditional probabilities. The prior probability is the probability which is based on our knowledge of the person's previous family, whereas the conditional probability is the probability that a person may be affected according to the age of the patient or the result of various tests which have been carried out (Emery, 1969 and 1979).

Autosomal dominant disorders include facioscapulohumeral muscular dystrophy, Huntington's chorea, myotonia congenita, neurofibromatosis and peroneal muscular atrophy. Provided the gene for a disorder is fully penetrant the probability of a person heterozygous for an autosomal dominant gene having any of his children affected is 50 per cent, and any unaffected children have no chance of passing on the disorder. With incomplete penetrance the situation is more difficult and careful clinical examination may be necessary to establish that the individual is clinically normal. With peroneal muscular atrophy sometimes individuals are clinically normal but have slowing of nerve conduction velocity. Autosomal recessive disorders include Friedreich's ataxia, limb girdle muscle atrophy, Refsum's syndrome and Werdnig–Hoffmann disease. In this situation unless the condition has developed as a new mutation both parents of an affected individual must be heterozygotes and the chance of such parents having an affected child is 1 in 4. Unless the recessive disease is very common it seldom appears in more than one generation and the probability of a carrier having affected children is very small unless they should marry a close relative. X-linked disorders include Duchenne and Becker muscular dystrophy. Duchenne dystrophy is a severe dystrophy in which males seldom live long enough to marry. A carrier female has a probability that half her daughters will be carriers and half her sons will be affected. Detection of carriers of Duchenne dystrophy is assisted by the fact that more than two-thirds have an elevated serum creatine kinase. Other aspects of genetic counselling include the detection of chromosome abnormalities and the antenatal recognition of congenital abnormalities such as Down's syndrome which is recognised by detecting chromosomal abnormality in the amniotic fluid. In open spina bifida the level of α-fetoprotein is elevated both in the blood stream and in the amniotic fluid. A raised level in the blood stream, however, is not diagnostic; but blood examination provides a useful screening test which can be carried out prior to amniocentesis.

REFERENCES

Basmajian, J V (1979) *Biofeedback – Principles and Practice for Clinicians*. The Williams and Wilkins Co., Baltimore.

Beecher, H K (1968) A definition of irreversible coma. Report of the Ad Hoc Committee of the Harvard Medical School to examine the Definition of Death. *Journal of the American Medical Association*, **205**, 337–339.

Caronna, J J, Levy, D E, Bates, D, Cartlidge, N E F, Knill-Jones, R P, Shaw, D A and Plum, F (1978) A prospective study of the neurological outcome of medical coma, in Neurology. In: *Proceedings of the 11th World Congress of Neurology, Amsterdam*, pp. 260–282. (Eds) W A Hartog-Jager, G W Bruyn and A P J Heijstee. Excerpta Medica, Amsterdam and Oxford.

Conference of Medical Royal Colleges (1976) Diagnosis of brain death. *British Medical Journal*, **2**, 1187–1188; *Lancet*, **2**, 1069–1071.

Emery, A E H (1969) Genetic counselling. *Scottish Medical Journal*, **14**, 335–347.

Emery, A E H (1979) *Elements of Medical Genetics*, 5th Edn. Churchill Livingstone, Edinburgh and London.

Glaser, G H (1978) Brain death. In: *Recent Advances in Clinical Neurology*. (Eds) W B Matthews and G H Glaser. Churchill Livingstone, Edinburgh and London.

International Federation of Societies for Electroencephalography and Clinical Neurophysiology (1974) Proceedings of the General Assembly. *Electroencephalography and Clinical Neurophysiology*, **37**, 521—553.

Jennett, B and Plum, F (1972) Persistent vegetative state after brain damage. *Lancet*, **1**, 734—737.

Jennet, B, Teasdale, G, Braakman, R, Minderhood, J, Heiden, J and Kurze, T (1978) Predicting outcome after severe head injury. In: *Proceedings of the 11th World Congress of Neurology, Amsterdam*, pp. 242—254. (Eds) W A Hartog-Jager, G W Bruyn and A P J Heijstee. Excerpta Medica, Amsterdam/Oxford.

Korein, J (1978) Terminology, definitions and usage. In: *Brain Death: Interrelated Medical and Social Issues*. (Ed) J Korein. *Annals of the New York Academy of Sciences*, **315**, 6—10.

Kutt, H, Brennan, R and McDouell, F (1968) Inhibition of diphenylhydantoin metabolism in rats and in rat liver microsomes by anti-tubercular drugs. *Neurology (Minneapolis)*, **18**, 706—714.

Plum, F and Posner, J B (1972) *The Diagnosis of Stupor and Coma*, 2nd Edn. F A Davis Co., Philadelphia.

Posner, J B (1978) Coma and other states of consciousness: the differential diagnosis of brain death. In: *Brain Death: Interrelated Medical and Social Issues*. (Ed) J Korein. *Annals of the New York Academy of Sciences*, **315**, 215—227.

Teasdale, G and Jennett, B (1974) Assessment of coma and impaired consciousness. *Lancet*, **2**, 81—83.

CHAPTER TWO

The Epilepsies and Disorders of Sleep

Seizures arise from a wide variety of structural and metabolic disorders affecting the brain. As the mechanisms contributing to their production, spread and termination are complex it is not surprising that the modes of action of various treatments are poorly understood. Various attempts have been made to classify these disorders into coherent logical groupings. The International Classification of the Epilepsies is the most comprehensive attempt, in which the epilepsies are grouped according to clinical seizure types, age, EEG findings, postulated anatomical substrate, and aetiology. A simpler classification into four groups is used in this chapter.

(1) Primary generalised seizures. These usually start in childhood or adolescence, and the discharges involve the thalamus and brainstem together with the cerebral cortex bilaterally. This group includes major seizures with tonic and clonic features, and petit mal or absence attacks. In the latter the clinical features, EEG appearances and response to anticonvulsants differ from grand mal seizures.

(2) Seizures with focal cortical origin. These arise most commonly in the temporal lobe and adjacent structures giving rise to the amazingly diverse manifestations of temporal lobe epilepsy (complex partial seizures). Simpler seizures with either motor, sensory or visual symptoms may arise from frontal, parietal or occipital cortex.

(3) Seizures with a focal origin and secondary generalised spread. These arise from a focal cortical lesion but secondary bilateral sychrony occurs.

(4) A complex mixture of cortical and subcortical attacks. These patients often have severe brain damage.

DIAGNOSIS

A clear diagnosis is essential before advice can be given about the prognosis, school, work, driving etc. and also for the selection of appropriate drug treatment. It is the clinical description of the attacks, either by the patient or by witnesses, that is the most important basis for making this diagnosis. In addition to having as full an account of the attacks as possible it is important to consider the patient's age and the circumstances of the seizures. They may occur during sleep, during awakening, or when awake. There may be a relationship to drug or alcohol withdrawal, stress, fever, or the menstrual cycle. Specific environmental stimuli such as flashing lights or other more complex stimuli may be important triggers. The clinical assessment should include consideration of the non-neurological causes of blackouts, e.g. cardiac arrhythmias, syncope, hyperventilation, and hysteria. A structural cause of the seizures should be identified, if possible. The appropriate investigations may range from none after a single, clearly described brief febrile convulsion to prolonged EEG or ECG recordings if the nature of the attacks are in doubt. Extensive metabolic or radiological studies may be indicated if the cause of the seizures is unclear.

EEG Studies

The value of EEG recordings is often poorly understood by the non-specialist. A standard EEG recording may be useful in several ways in the assessment of epilepsy. In young patients with brief lapses of consciousness which may be 'petit mal', 3-per-second spike and wave activity on the EEG may be clearly distinguished from brief focal temporal lobe discharges and from minor atypical generalised seizures. The EEG may confirm photosensitivity and occasionally a generalised or focal seizure itself is recorded. An EEG recording may identify a consistent focal abnormality that requires further investigation for lesions such as a tumour or an arteriovenous malformation. There are, however, important limitations in the use of EEG recordings. Firstly, as some patients with undoubted focal or generalised seizures may have normal standard EEG recordings, a normal recording does not preclude epilepsy. Special techniques of recording such as the use of sphenoidal electrodes, prolonged telemetry or tape-recordings, or the enhancement of paroxysmal activity with sleep or bemegride increases the number of abnormalities. These techniques are time-consuming and are not to be routinely used. The second limitation is that focal and generalised paroxysmal activity can be recorded from some subjects who have never had seizures, particularly if there is a family history of epilepsy. Therefore discharges on an EEG do not make a diagnosis of epilepsy. Furthermore, the presence of paroxysmal activity in the EEG is not a reliable guide to the prognosis, except perhaps in 3-per-second spike and wave activity.

Other investigations

It is commonly asked how far investigations should be taken in the common situation of a child or adolescent with the recent onset of seizures. Such patients should have an EEG. Skull X-rays are usually normal but the abnormalities that are occasionally revealed, such as intracranial calcification and pituitary fossa changes, are particularly important. CT scanning is seldom helpful in this age range. In the older patients investigations may have to be extensive, including CT scanning.

GENERAL ADVICE

The physician must be prepared to discuss the diagnosis and management with patients and relatives as they are likely to be anxious and in need of explanations and advice. Misconceptions are still common — not only in the general public, including teachers and employers, but in patients and their relatives. The advice and the discussion may include the avoidance of factors which increase seizures in some patients such as photic stimulation, stress, or the abuse of alcohol. Patients will be concerned about the implications of epilepsy for work, driving, school and sport, and also about the genetic influences and the prognosis for recovery.

Factors modifying the occurrence of seizures

1. *Reflex epilepsies*

Photogenic seizures are the commonest of the reflex epilepsies. About 5 per cent of patients with epilepsy are sensitive to stimulation by light, and in these a common trigger is watching television. As some patients who are not photosensitive may have seizures fortuitously while watching television, the EEG is useful in confirming photoconvulsive responses. If a photosensitive patient has seizures only while watching TV it may be possible to prevent further attacks without anticonvulsants by simple advice. The intensity of the photic stimuli should be reduced by viewing in a room with adequate background illumination and reduced screen brightness. Viewing from close to the screen should be avoided as it increases the intensity of the stimulus and may permit perception of flicker at 25 Hz (30 Hz in the USA) which is a more potent trigger for seizures than the normal frequency of 50 or 60 Hz. Adjustment of flickering screens by the patient should be avoided. When approaching the television set one eye should be closed or covered because monocular occlusion usually prevents the attacks. The use of one polaroid lens with a polaroid sheet in front of the screen has been suggested but this should be unnecessary. Complete avoidance of television is unlikely to be acceptable in our addicted societies.

Seizures induced by other visual stimuli such as reading, pattern, colour, by auditory stimuli (sudden noise, music) or somatosensory stimulation may be treated by conditioning methods (Forster, 1972). As the numbers of patients are relatively small, and the techniques are time-consuming and unpredictable in their results, they have not been widely used. Some patients with focal motor or sensory seizures find that the attacks may be inhibited by a specific activity like moving or rubbing a limb.

2. *Emotion, arousal and stress*

Although in some patients stress or emotion clearly exacerbates or precipitates seizures, the prevention of these attacks by altering the patient's mental or emotional state is limited to a small group of patients. An approach by behavioural therapy has been described (Mostofsky, 1977) but further clinical experience needs to be reported. Perhaps the most widely applicable simple measure arises from the recognition that seizures are more common when the patient is tired or bored, and that stimulating but not over-demanding activity reduces seizures. EEG recordings have shown that the frequency of spike-and-wave activity is less with arousal and more with inactivity (Bureau *et al.*, 1968). The practical implication is that patients are better when active at school, work and recreation, but worse when inactive in an undemanding perhaps over-protected environment. This has important implications for advice on work, school and leisure activities, as will be discussed subsequently.

Implications of epilepsy for daily activities

1. *School*

Most epileptic children attend normal schools and some do not have attacks at school. Problems may arise at school for various reasons and each possibility needs consideration.

(a) Lack of information. It is usually best that teachers know about the epilepsy. They can then handle problems sensibly in the class and explain the disorder in an appropriate manner to classmates. The well-informed teacher then becomes a key person in the management at school. Information may go to the school from the patient's physician, the school doctor, the parents, and leaflets or books.

(b) Unrecognised attacks. Absence or temporal lobe attacks may be unrecognised or misinterpreted as stupidity, laziness, dyslexia or behaviour problems, and may explain some difficulties at schools. Prolonged EEG monitoring may reveal paroxysmal activity which is missed by the parents, teachers, or a standard EEG recording.

(c) Drug effects. As anticonvulsants may interfere with attention and learning (reviewed by Trimble and Reynolds, 1976) it is important to select less-sedative anticonvulsants. In patients with refractory seizures the occurrence of some attacks may have to be accepted. These may be preferable to marked toxic effects from the drugs.

(d) Behavioural problems. These may occur in epileptic children, as in others, and careful assessment of the individual circumstances is needed. Difficult behaviour may arise from different causes such as inept or over-protective handling at home, rejection by peers, subclinical or overt seizures, adverse effects of drugs, or the presence of associated brain lesions.

(e) Organic brain damage. Some patients with right temporal lobe lesions may have subtle defects of visuo-spacial memory, while left-sided temporal lobe lesions may produce minor alteration in language function. Other types of brain damage may result in mental retardation with emotional immaturity, hyperkinetic states, hemiplegia or involuntary movement disorders. The more severely affected children are better educated in special schools where the specific difficulties of the child can be managed. These special schools may also help some patients with severe behavioural problems without additional neurological deficits.

2. *Sport, including swimming*

A rigid prohibition of sport, particularly swimming and cycling, is now giving way to more permissive advice for two reasons. Firstly, it emerges that the risks are small in the adequately controlled epileptic, perhaps because of the arousal discussed earlier. Indeed, supervised swimming is encouraged in some special schools for children with epilepsy where, even in this population, attacks seldom occur. 'Contact' sports such as football in which there are minor blows to the head are not associated with increased seizures (Livingstone and Berman, 1973). The second reason for changing the attitudes to sport is to avoid the psychological consequences of an isolated and over-protected childhood. The seizures may disappear but the disturbed personality persists. Obviously, if the patient is having frequent fits then potentially dangerous sports should be avoided at that time, but every effort should be made to encourage as normal a life as possible.

3. *Work*

The person with epilepsy should be encouraged to take up as normal and satisfying work as possible and indeed the majority of patients hold jobs in open competition and work well. Driving is precluded in many patients and this limits the choice of occupations. It is sensible that particularly dangerous jobs, such as working at heights or with hazardous machinery, should be avoided. In some patients it is not the epilepsy but the personality that makes obtaining work difficult. These personality problems can arise from educational, social and emotional difficulties, some of which originate in poor early management.

Patients often ask whether they should reveal the diagnosis to employers, and a general answer cannot be given. Some employers may be ignorant and therefore prejudiced about epilepsy. Job applications may be helped by a medical statement which avoids only stating that the patient suffers from epilepsy but indicates in addition the type and frequency of attacks so that the prospective employer may have a better understanding of the problems. In the UK, if the patient cannot find employment, the help of the Disablement Rehabilitation Officer (DRO) should be sought, for he can assess the work potential and advise on possible opportunities. Some patients may find employment easier to obtain when on the Disablement Register. If employment still cannot be found, particularly if there are additional neurological deficits, then sheltered employment is needed.

4. *Driving*

Each country has somewhat different legislation concerning driving by persons with epilepsy. In the UK, according to the Road Traffic Act of 1974, patients may only drive provided they have been free of fits for at least 3 years or have an established pattern of nocturnal attacks for 3 years and that his/her driving is not likely to be a danger to the public. The doctor should explain the law to the patient but in the UK, unlike some countries, there is no legal requirement to inform the authorities. The regulations for driving heavy goods and public service vehicles are more rigid. All persons who have had epileptic attacks after the age of 3 are precluded from holding such a licence.

The legislation is clear for most situations but where it is uncertain the best advice on this subject is to be found in The Royal Commission on Accident Prevention (1976). The commonest problems arise in the patient with a single seizure and in the patient with attacks on drug withdrawal. If an isolated seizure has occurred with a precipitant that is unlikely to recur then this should not be considered as epilepsy with the implication of a liability to recurrent seizures. In this situation, and where the cause of a blackout is uncertain, private driving should be suspended for 6–12 months, but HGV and PSV licences will be revoked. A clear unprovoked seizure associated with EEG abnormalities may be considered as the onset of epilepsy and the 3-year rule obtains. If seizures occur in an adolescent when withdrawing medication under medical advice, it is reasonable that driving should be permitted after 6 months provided that the patient returns to the dose that had previously prevented seizures for over 3 years. Patients should be warned that they should remain on the anticonvulsant dose that has been effective, and that driving should be suspended if the treatment is changed. They should also receive explanations that alcohol may interact with their medication, in addition to the usual hazards of drink and driving, and that undue exhaustion increases the liability to seizures.

The accident rate is reported in some studies to be slightly increased in epileptic patients but the total contribution of epilepsy to the accident rate is only in the region of 1–3 per 10 000 accidents. One study, however, which included epileptics who had not declared their driving to the licensing authorities has reported a lower accident rate than in the control population (Laks and Korczyn, 1977).

5. *Genetic factors*

Patients are often concerned about the risk that epilepsy may be inherited. A familial factor does emerge from a number of studies. Briefly, the concordance rates for uniovular twins is higher than for binovular ones, and the prevalence of epilepsy or EEG abnormalities is greater in the families of patients who have had febrile convulsions, petit mal or idiopathic epilepsy than in control populations. There is, in addition, evidence that genetic factors may predispose to the occurrence of temporal lobe epilepsy and seizures occurring after head injury.

For genetic counselling the risks can be stated only in broad terms. When the mother is epileptic the risk of having a child that develops epilepsy is increased from about 0.5 per cent to a higher risk, variously reported as between 2 and 6 per cent. The risks are higher for mothers with idiopathic than 'acquired' epilepsies. The risk is considerably increased if both parents are epileptic. Whether families consider these risks to be too high is a personal matter, but most families gain some reassurance that the risks are relatively low, and that limitation of family size is not indicated when a single parent is epileptic.

PROGNOSIS

The prognosis depends mainly on the age and type of seizure.

(a) Febrile convulsions

Less than 5 per cent of patients with brief typical febrile convulsions subsequently develop epilepsy. The risk is greater in patients with prolonged febrile convulsions which may result in hippocampal damage. The risk of recurrent febrile convulsions is higher with patients less than 19 months old, in those with previous febrile convulsions, a family history of epilepsy, or a pre-existing neurological abnormality.

(b) Petit mal

About 80 per cent of patients with petit mal only cease to have attacks within 5 years. If other types of seizures also occur then the prognosis is poorer. If grand mal is also present 50 per cent of patients cease having petit mal at 5 years, and an even smaller number spontaneously remit if akinetic attacks and myoclonus are also present.

(c) A single generalised seizure

A single attack in a young person does not make a diagnosis of epilepsy but the risk of having further attacks is uncertain. If the attack was related to a lack of sleep, emotional or physical stress the prognosis is good in that few patients have further unprovoked attacks. In one series only 2 of 37 such patients subsequently had unprovoked seizures (Friis and Lund, 1974). In another study, 39 per cent of men in the US Navy presenting with single seizures had no further attacks at follow-up. If the attack was a clearly described grand mal convulsion, if there was post-ictal confusion or an abnormal EEG the prognosis was poorer (Johnson *et al.*, 1972).

(d) Recurrent grand mal attacks

The prognosis is worse for patients with attacks over a prolonged period, those with underlying brain lesions, low IQ, or additional focal attacks.

(e) Partial (focal) epilepsies

Focal seizures are less likely to disappear than generalised ones. The remission rate for temporal lobe seizures was reported as low as 20—35 per cent (Rodin, 1968). The benign focal epilepsy of childhood with Rolandic or mid-temporal spikes usually disappears in adolescence. One important recent study of children with temporal lobe epilepsy helps to give a clearer prognosis. About one-third of children subsequently become seizure-free, about one-third become independent but remain on anticonvulsants, and one-third remain dependent, living with parents or in an institution. Poor prognostic factors are low IQ, the onset of seizures before 28 months, five or more grand mal seizures as well as temporal lobe attacks, frequent temporal lobe attacks, a left-sided focus, hyperkinesis, episodes of severe rage, and a need for special schooling (Lindsay *et al.*, 1979). Boys with attacks persisting into adolescence lack sexual drive. In adolescence, if seizures have ceased and there are few poor prognostic factors, anticonvulsant therapy should be withdrawn. If seizures continue despite anticonvulsant drugs then temporal lobectomy may be considered.

ANTICONVULSANT DRUGS

The improvements in the management of the epilepsies in recent years has come largely from wiser use of established anticonvulsants and the introduction of newer ones. Although the pharmacokinetics of anticonvulsant drugs are more fully known, their mode of action is still poorly understood. In the next section important drugs are discussed individually, and in the subsequent section consideration is given to the selection of drugs for particular clinical situations. The use of drugs in neonatal and early childhood epilepsy is not discussed.

PHENYTOIN

Phenytoin (5,6-diphenyl hydantoin) is the most widely used of a group of hydantoins with anticonvulsant properties.

Absorption and administration

Phenytoin is mainly absorbed in the small intestine and reaches a peak serum level after a single oral dose in 3—12 h. The extent of this absorption can be critical, as discussed later, when the metabolism of the drug is approaching saturation. In this situation a small increase in absorption, such as that which may occur with the change in formulation of the drug from a calcium sulphate to a sodium salt, may result in intoxication.

Intramuscular phenytoin is precipitated in a relatively insoluble form in muscle and its absorption into the circulation is therefore delayed. Therefore i.m. phenytoin is not suitable for the treatment of status epilepticus. The marked reduction in absorption from muscle is illustrated by a suggested regime for changing from oral to i.m. phenytoin for a short period of surgery. It was recommended that the i.m. phenytoin dose be 50 per cent higher than the oral dose but that on a return to an oral regime the phenytoin dose should be half the original dose for the same period of time that the patient received i.m. administration (Wilder *et al.*, 1974).

Phenytoin is produced in an alkaline solvent for i.v. infusion. This may cause venospasm and thrombophlebitis unless given into a fast-running drip. The phenytoin is likely to precipitate out if added to saline or other i.v. infusions. It is therefore best given as a bolus injection into an i.v. drip. The rate of injection should not exceed 50 mg/min to prevent cardiac adverse effects. The dose is 150—250 mg but if status epilepticus continues in the subsequent 30 min a further 100—150 mg may be given.

Distribution

Phenytoin is over 90 per cent bound to plasma and it is the unbound, largely ionised fraction that is rapidly distributed to the tissues, including the brain. Most assays measure the total phenytoin, except for salivary estimations which reflect the unbound fraction. Serum binding is important in diseases in which the plasma proteins are reduced, e.g. the nephrotic syndrome. In these disorders toxicity may occur from high free phenytoin concentrations although the total phenytoin is not elevated. Furthermore, drugs which displace phenytoin from binding sites, e.g. salicylic acid, phenylbutazone, sulphafurazole, increase the free phenytoin concentrations.

Metabolism

Two pharmacokinetic findings are important in the wise use of phenytoin. Firstly, individuals differ widely in their rate of metabolism of phenytoin, and secondly, saturation kinetics occur in the therapeutic range. Phenytoin is hydroxylated in the liver. The metabolite is excreted into bile, reabsorbed in the small intestine and excreted in the urine. As less than 5 per cent of phenytoin is excreted unchanged in the urine, renal failure does not result in marked changes in plasma levels. Individuals who metabolise phenytoin slowly may be adequately treated with 200 mg daily, while rapid metabolisers may need in excess of 500 mg daily. Children usually hydroxylate phenytoin rapidly. The saturation kinetics are most clearly illustrated in Figure 2.1. This shows the differences in rates of metabolism in five different patients, and also the non-linear relationship between dose and plasma level. With increasing doses of phenytoin the hepatic enzyme systems become saturated and the serum levels start to rise rapidly. Unfortunately these changes start occurring when the serum levels are in the 'therapeutic' range. At this stage small increases in the bioavailability of the drug or displacement from plasma-binding sites cause large changes in free phenytoin levels. Because such marked changes in serum levels may occur with small changes in the dose, the manufacturers of phenytoin have introduced 50 mg and 25 mg capsules to allow a finer adjustment of serum levels in some patients.

The half-life varies considerably from 9 to 140 h, commonly about 24 h. Therefore a plateau level is not generally reached until 4—5 days after a change in dose.

Serum levels and dosages

In recent years the serum levels have become standard assays for they provide a useful guide to treatment. The 'therapeutic' or 'optimal' range of serum levels is that at which seizure control is most likely to occur without undue adverse effects. The range for phenytoin is 40—80 μmol/l (10—20 μg/ml). Serum level measurements are useful in patients with refractory seizures where a low level may arise from non-compliance or rapid metabolism. These patients should not be considered as treatment failures until an adequate serum level has been obtained. The assays are

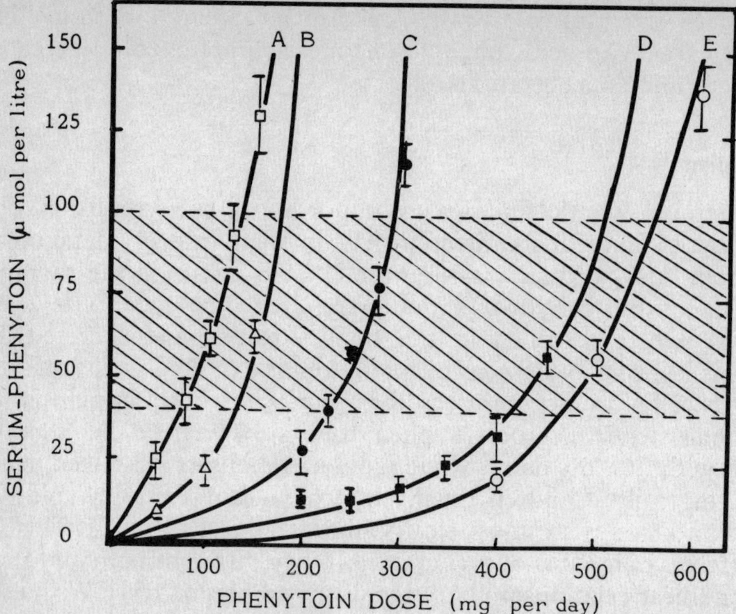

Figure 2.1   Relation between daily dose of phenytoin and resulting serum level in five patients on several different doses of the drug.

Each point represents the mean of three to eight separate estimations in the steady state. The bars represent 1 SEM. The hatched area represents the therapeutic range of serum levels. The curves were fitted by computer, using the Michaelis—Menten equation.

(1 μmol/l = 0.25 μg/ml.) Richens and Dunlop, 1975. Reproduced by kind permission of A Richens and the Editor of *The Lancet*

also very helpful where drug intoxication is suspected, particularly if more than one anticonvulsant is being used. The serum level estimations are a guide to treatment and the physician should not feel it obligatory that all patients have 'therapeutic' levels. Some patients have complete control of seizures with serum levels below this range, while others may have unacceptable sedation within the therapeutic range and a few are relatively free of adverse effects with levels above the upper end of the range. In paediatric practice salivary level estimations are useful because venepunctures are avoided.

A convenient starting dose in adults is 300 mg daily. This may be given as a single daily dose but as many patients may forget occasional doses, it is often preferable to give it in two doses. Some patients may require as much as 600 mg daily. The recommended dosage in children

Table 2.1 A regime for starting phenytoin and phenobarbitone in children (Richens, 1976)

Body-weight (kg)	Phenytoin dose		Phenobarbitone dose	
	mg/kg	Total dose (mg/day)*	mg/kg	Total dose (mg/day)*
6—10	10.0	100	4.5	45
11—15	9.0	125	4.0	60
16—20	8.0	150	3.5	60
21—25	7.0	175	3.0	75
26—30	6.5	200	2.5	75
31—35	5.5	200	2.5	90
36—40	5.5	225	2.0	90
41—45	5.5	250	2.0	90
46—50	5.0	250	2.0	100
51—60	5.0	300	2.0	120

* Doses rounded off to suit Epanutin Infatabs (50 mg scored tablets), and phenobarbitone 15 mg, 30 mg, 60 mg and 100 mg tablets.

is shown in Table 2.1. It is better given in tablet or capsule form, if possible, for the suspension needs to be carefully shaken before administration lest a variable dose be given.

For a rapid increase in serum levels an oral phenytoin loading regime may be used. A dose of about 20 mg/kg over 6—12 h produces serum levels in the therapeutic range rapidly in many patients (Record *et al.*, 1979).

Drug interactions

Important drug interactions may occur from either the induction or the impairment of the hepatic metabolism of phenytoin. The biotransformation of phenytoin may be inhibited by disulfiram or sulthiame, thereby increasing the half-life and elevating the serum levels. In contrast, the enzyme systems may be induced by ethanol or by carbamazepine. Phenobarbitone has an unpredictable effect for it is a potent inducer of the hydroxylase systems but it also competes with phenytoin for these enzymes. The net result may, therefore, be an increase, a decrease or little change in phenytoin level. Table 2.2 shows the drugs

Table 2.2 Drug interactions with phenytoin

Drugs increasing phenytoin levels	*Drugs decreasing phenytoin levels*
Phenobarbitone	Phenobarbitone
Sulthiame	Carbamazepine
Isoniazid	Ethanol
Chloramphenicol	Diazepam
Dicoumarol	Clonazepam
Pheneturide	
Disulfiram	
Methylphenidate	
Chlordiazepoxide/diazepam	

that significantly affect phenytoin levels. In addition, phenytoin may alter the metabolism of other drugs and some hormones (Table 2.3). One worrying report for the management of young women on phenytoin is that the metabolism of oral contraceptives may be so enhanced that pregnancy may result. The risk is likely to be small but low dose contraceptives should be avoided in patients on anticonvulsant therapy. The increase in vitamin D_3 metabolism is the basis for the long-term bone complications.

Mechanism of action

Despite much research in recent years phenytoin's mode of action is still poorly understood. A clear explanation might be most illuminating in the study of epilepsy. There is evidence that phenytoin inhibits the spread of seizures, that it acts in part *via* the cerebellum and the spinal cord, that it affects 5-HT systems, and that at a cellular level it alters ATPase systems.

Table 2.3 Drugs having concentrations reduced by phenytoin

Warfarin	Phenylbutazone
Coumarins	Antipyrine
Phenothiazines	Cortisol
Tricyclic drugs	Dexamethasone
Doxycycline	Oral contraceptives
Digitoxin	Vitamin D_3
Quinine and quinidine	

Adverse effects

The commonest complications of phenytoin treatment are in the nervous system and the skin.

(a) Nervous system

Slight drowsiness and slowing of thought may occur within the 'therapeutic' range although these effects are less prominent than with phenobarbitone. The onset may be so insidious that the patient only recognises the impairment after drug withdrawal. Higher doses result in a more severe encephalopathy with drowsiness, mental slowing and impaired concentration and drive. Occasionally a paradoxical increase in seizures may occur and the risk is that these seizures are misinterpreted and more phenytoin given, thereby exacerbating the intoxication.

A cerebellar syndrome consisting of ataxia, inco-ordination of the hands, dysarthria and a nystagmus may develop. This is usually reversible although there has been some evidence that irreversible Purkinje cell damage may occur.

Less commonly, a reversible involuntary movement disorder consisting of choreoathetosis or dystonia may occur. Other occasional effects are a mild sensory neuropathy (rarely severe) or intermittent diplopia.

(b) Skin problems

These are common, with acne, hursutism, and slight coarsening of the facial features. These may particularly embarrass young female patients and may be considered as an argument against using phenytoin in this group. Rashes and the Stevens—Johnson syndrome may also occur.

(c) Gum hypertrophy

Hypertrophy of the gums occurs in about 10 per cent of patients and is commoner with high phenytoin levels, poor dental hygiene and IgA deficiency.

(d) Gastrointestinal side-effects

These comprise nausea, vomiting, and, uncommonly, constipation. When the nausea and vomiting is combined with CNS intoxication the clinical picture may be mistaken for a serious expanding intracranial lesion and quite inappropriate investigations may be done. Hepatitis may occur.

(e) Folate deficiency

Folate deficiency may arise with phenytoin and barbiturates. The increased utilisation of folate as a cofactor in the hydroxylation of these anticonvulsants occasionally results in megaloblastic anaemia, a peripheral neuropathy or an encephalopathy. The role of folate in the control of seizures has been controversial. Early reports that the treatment of folate deficiency improves the encephalopathy but worsens the seizures have not been consistently confirmed (Reynolds, 1973). The improvement with folate treatment may have occurred because the folate permits an increased rate of hydroxylation of phenytoin, a fall in serum level, and therefore a decrease in adverse effects. As folate deficiency only develops in some patients with long-term treatment it is wise to treat only these patients (10 mg daily) rather than to give folate prophylactically.

Other rare haematological effects of phenytoin are aplastic anaemia, agranulocytosis and thrombocytopenia.

(f) Metabolic effects

Many metabolic effects have been described but their clinical importance is uncertain. Inhibition of insulin release, the altered hypothalamic control of the pituitary gland, displacement of thyroxine from plasma-binding sites, and the enhancement of the conversion of thyroxine to tri-iodothyronine may occur. The induction of vitamin D metabolism results in osteomalacia but this is usually biochemical and not symptomatic. Symptomatic patients require treatment with supplementary vitamin D.

(g) Immunological systems

Immunological systems are occasionally affected. IgA deficiency occurs in some patients (Aarli, 1976) and it appears that it develops in patients with pre-treatment concentrations at the lower end of the normal range. A lupus erythematosus-like syndrome, lymphadenopathy, or a pseudolymphoma occasionally occurs but these may be idiosyncratic reactions and the overall risk of developing a phenytoin-induced immune disorder is low.

BARBITURATES

Although phenobarbitone and primidone are still widely used, there has been a decline in their popularity, mainly due to their adverse effects.

Phenobarbitone

Pharmacokinetics

Phenobarbitone is readily absorbed from the gastrointestinal tract, mainly the small intestine, reaching a peak level 1—6 h after administration. As a similar time is required for the peak plasma level after i.m. administration phenobarbitone is unsuitable for the treatment of status epilepticus. The plasma binding is relatively low at about 50 per cent and therefore drug interactions with phenobarbitone binding are seldom important. Administered phenobarbitone is widely distributed in the body. It is hydroxylated in the liver but as this is not saturable in the therapeutic range, unlike phenytoin, increments in the dose produce a linear increase in plasma level. It is a potent enzyme-inducer, increasing the metabolism of coumarins, warfarin, digitoxin, chlorpromazine, vitamin D and cortisol in the liver. As stated earlier the interaction with phenytoin is complex, resulting sometimes in increased, unchanged, or reduced phenytoin levels.

Serum levels and dosages

The therapeutic range is 60—160 μmol/l (15—40 μg/ml). Treatment may be started in adults with 60 mg daily, with gradual increments to 180 mg daily if necessary. The dosage for children is shown in Table 2.1. The half-life is 53—140 h in adults, shorter in children, and therefore a single daily dose is satisfactory. A plateau level may not be achieved for up to 3 weeks after a change in dose and therefore serum level estimations taken earlier may be misleading.

Adverse effects

Drowsiness is common in therapeutic doses and is an important reason for the growing preference for newer anticonvulsants. It may be avoided, at least in part, by gradual increments in dosage, and it may diminish with time. The finding of impairment on psychological testing supports the description of impaired mental function given by patients or relatives.

An important adverse effect in some children is the development of irritability, belligerence and hyperactivity. Ataxia, inco-ordination, and nystagmus may occur.

As with phenytoin the barbiturates may cause folate deficiency, rashes, skin changes, and osteomalacia.

Primidone (Mysoline)

Primidone is rapidly absorbed with a mean peak level after 3 h (range 0.5—9 h) and it is metabolised in the liver to various metabolites, the most important of which are phenobarbitone and phenylethylmelonamide (PEMA). Both primidone and these metabolites have anticonvulsant effects. Correlation of the serum level with the clinical response is difficult because of the different half-lives of primidone and its metabolites (primidone about 6—7 h, PEMA 24—48 h and phenobarbitone 53—140 h). Primidone and PEMA are only slightly bound to plasma and therefore interaction with other drugs by displacement from binding sites is not important. In renal failure the dosage may have to be reduced as both primidone and PEMA are excreted by the kidneys to a greater extent than phenobarbitone.

Some individuals exhibit a marked sensitivity to primidone with the development of drowsiness, vertigo and a sense of intoxication within an hour of taking it. The starting dose in adults should therefore be low at 125 mg, with increments thereafter every 3—4 days to an effective dosage range which is usually 750—1500 mg daily. For children aged 1—2 years the dosage is 250—500 mg daily, at 2—5 years the dosage is 500—750 mg daily, and for 6—9 year-old children the dosage is 750—1000 mg daily.

The adverse effects are similar to those found with phenobarbitone.

CARBAMAZEPINE

Carbamazepine, marketed as Tegretol, is an iminostilbene, chemically related to tricyclic antidepressants, but its mode of action is unknown. It is effective for major convulsions and focal seizures.

Pharmacokinetics

The peak level is reached after oral administration in about 2½ h, with 70—80 per cent binding to plasma. Carbamazepine is metabolised in part to an epoxide but there are several other metabolites. One important observation for management is that it induces its own metabolism and therefore increasing doses may be needed in the early weeks of treatment.

Serum level and dosage

Carbamazepine is formulated in 100 mg and 200 mg tablets, and in a syrup with 100 mg/5 ml. It has a half-life of 8½–19 h and the daily requirement may be divided into two, three or four doses. The timing of a previous dose should be considered when interpreting the serum level.

The dosage required is very variable, from 300 mg to about 2000 mg daily in adults, with the majority requiring 600–1200 mg daily. The dosage in children is 200–400 mg daily at 1–5 years, 400–600 mg at 5–10 years, and 600–1000 mg at 10–15 years. The therapeutic range of serum levels is 16–40 μmol/l (4–10 μg/ml) but carbamazepine may be effective in some patients below these levels.

Adverse effects

Drowsiness, dizziness and ataxia may occur, particularly in the elderly. The mental effects have been the source of much controversy as elevation of mood with improved alertness and concentration may occur on changing from phenytoin or barbiturates to carbamazepine. It seems likely that these 'psychotropic' effects arise simply in comparison with the more sedative drugs rather than from inherent beneficial effects of carbamazepine on mood and mental processes. Some patients develop dyskinetic eye movements with or without ataxia, 1–2 h after a dose.

Aplastic anaemia is very uncommon and has been reported in the elderly taking carbamazepine for the treatment of trigeminal neuralgia. Progressive slight decline in white cell concentration may occur over several years, and occasionally there is leucopenia. A mild generalised rash, a light-sensitive dermatitis and the Stevens–Johnson syndrome have been reported. An ADH-like effect may result in hyponatraemia, decreased osmolality, and impairment of water excretion (Perucca *et al.*, 1978). Clinical effects of this hyponatraemia may develop, but usually when the serum level is within the toxic range.

SODIUM VALPROATE

Sodium valproate is the sodium salt of dipropylacetic acid (valproic acid) and is marketed in the UK as 'Epilim'. In the USA valproic acid is sold as 'Depakene' (review, Bruni and Wilder, 1979). It has the merit of being effective against petit mal as well as generalised convulsions, and to a lesser extent focal seizures. Even less is known about its mode of action than about the other major anticonvulsants. The evidence that it impairs the metabolism of γ-aminobutyric acid (GABA), an inhibitory neurotransmitter, is based on experimental studies using high dosage and may not be relevant to its action in man. There is evidence that the anticonvulsant action after a single dose starts a few hours after the peak serum and may last for hours or even up to 5 days (Rowan *et al.*, 1979). These observations explain the poor correlation between serum levels and the clinical response (Wulff *et al.*, 1977).

Pharmacokinetics

Sodium valproate is readily absorbed with a peak plasma level at 1–4 h. The half-life is 8–15 h and it is excreted in the urine mainly as conjugates. A small fraction is oxidised to ketone bodies. The plasma binding is high at 84–95 per cent. As sodium valproate impairs the metabolism of phenobarbitone combined therapy may produce elevation of phenobarbitone levels and drowsiness. The interaction with phenytoin is less important. It may reduce the total phenytoin levels slightly but the concentration of free phenytoin is unchanged. Valproate may potentiate effects of monoamine oxidase inhibitors.

Serum levels and dosage

A therapeutic range of 300–600 μmol/l has been claimed but, because of the poor correlation between the serum levels and the clinical response, the value of these measurements is uncertain, except in assessing compliance.

In adults the starting dose is 200 mg t.i.d. with increments every 3–4 days, if necessary. Seizure control is most commonly achieved with a dosage in the range 600–1400 mg daily. Further increments up to 2500 mg daily may occasionally be required. In children under 20 kg a dose of 20–30 mg/kg should be given. Children over 20 kg may commence with 400 mg daily, with subsequent increments until control is achieved or adverse effects occur, usually in the range 20–30 mg/kg daily. Sodium valproate is formulated in 200 mg or 500 mg tablets or as a syrup but a formulation for parenteral use is not available. Recently enteric-coated formulations of both 500 mg and 200 mg doses have been produced and these may be used in patients with gastrointestinal adverse effects while taking the previous formulations. Rectal administration has been described for status epilepticus although it was not shown to produce rapid control of the seizures (Vajda *et al.*, 1978).

Adverse effects

Sodium valproate is relatively free of sedative side-effects. Like carbamazepine the question of a psychotrophic effect has been raised because of the improvement on changing from barbiturates and phenytoin. However, in a controlled trial a slight deterioration in psychomotor assessment was found (Sommerbeck *et al.*, 1977). Tremor or increased appetite and weight gain may occur. Nausea, retrosternal discomfort or diarrhoea may occur at the start of treatment. A reversible alopecia may occur which is usually mild and transient. Curiously, the hair may regrow curly. Slight elevation of hepatic enzymes may also occur. There have been a few cases of severe hepatitis and a few deaths attributed to valproic acid. Mild thrombocytopenia and interference with Factor VIII metabolism are reported.

ETHOSUXIMIDE

Ethosuximide, marketed as Zarontin, is used for the treatment of petit mal. Phensuximide and methsuximide are related drugs but the former is more toxic and the latter less effective than ethosuximide.

Pharmacokinetics

It is readily absorbed with a peak level in 1—4 h and is rapidly distributed to the tissues, including the brain. The half-life is 60—100 h in adults, and 16—68 h in children. Therefore a single daily dose may be suitable although many physicians prefer a divided dose regime. The plasma binding is negligible and drug interactions are not recognised to be important. Ethosuximide is metabolised in the liver by oxidation and conjugation to a glucuronide to produce three inactive metabolites. Only 10—20 per cent is excreted unchanged in the urine.

Serum levels and dosage

The best control of absence attacks occurs with the serum levels of 300—700 µmol/l (40—100 µg/ml). The serum level usually remains stable over several months.

Ethosuximide is formulated in 250 mg capsules or an elixir in a concentration of 250 mg/ml. In children a starting dose is 20 mg/kg, and increments should be at weekly intervals or more because of the long half-life.

Adverse effects

Mild side-effects such as nausea, drowsiness, dizziness or headache often disappear with continued treatment at the same dose. Skin rashes may occur. Behavioural manifestations with restlessness, hyperactivity, insomnia, impaired concentration, or aggressiveness seldom develop. Leucopenia and, rarely, pancytopenia have been reported.

BENZODIAZEPINES

The benzodiazepines have some anticonvulsant activity and the most important two are clonazepam and diazepam. Either drug may be used parenterally in status epilepticus, and oral clonazepam can be used in the control of petit mal and generalised convulsions. In addition nitrazepam orally has some anticonvulsant effects.

Clonazepam

Marketed as Rivotril, clonazepam achieves peak serum levels in 3—12 h after administration. The half-life after acute administration is 18—37 h, but after chronic treatment the metabolism is increased and the half-life falls to 8—29 h. Tolerance develops over several months.

Dosage

Serum level estimations are not in routine use. Clonazepam is formulated in 0.5 mg and 2 mg tablets. Oral treatment should start with a low dose, not greater than 1 mg daily in adults, 0.5 mg daily in children, and 0.25 mg daily in infants and small children. The oral dosage range in adults is 4—8 mg, in children of 5—12 years it is 3—6 mg, and in children of 1—3 years it is 1—3 mg daily. Because of the long half-life it may be given as a daily or twice-daily dose.

In status epilepticus adults should be given 1 mg (infants and small children 0.5 mg) in an i.v. bolus over about 30 s, repeated if the seizure is not controlled. Alternatively, it may be given by i.v. infusion with 3 mg freshly mixed with saline or dextrose solutions given over 12 h in adults.

Adverse effects

Drowsiness is the major adverse effect limiting the use of clonazepam. It may be avoided in part by the gradual introduction of therapy. In addition, inco-ordination, ataxia and hypotonia may occur. Paradoxically, agitation, irritability and inattention are other adverse effects. An unexpected adverse effect is a paradoxical increase in seizures of a variety of types (Browne and Penry, 1973). There is evidence that phenytoin metabolism may be impaired when the drugs are given concurrently.

Bronchial and salivary hypersecretion is potentially serious in infants and small children. Clonazepam is remarkably free from hepatic, haematological and skin complications.

Diazepam

This drug is now widely used in the treatment of status epilepticus and serial epilepsy. It acts rapidly when given by a bolus i.v. injection of 10 mg in adults or 0.15–0.25 mg/kg in children. This is given at a rate of about 2 mg/min in adults and older children, or 1 mg/min in children less than 5 years old. An alternative regime is to give a rapid injection of 0.5–2 mg over 5 s in children, repeated if necessary, to produce a rapid control of seizures without significant adverse effects (Pampiglione and Da Costa, 1975). The risk with rapid injections is depression or arrest of respiration, particularly when other anticonvulsants such as barbiturates have been used. Intravenous administration produces an earlier onset of effects than an intramuscular route and avoids the risk of delayed adverse effects if other anticonvulsants are given subsequently in refractory patients. Repeated 10 mg boluses, or an infusion of 50 mg in saline or dextrose over 12 h, may be given to adults. The maximum dose is 3 mg/kg body-weight over 24 h.

CHLORMETHIAZOLE

Chlormethiazole (Heminevrin) is derived from the thiazole moiety of the thiamine molecule. It may control status epilepticus given by an i.v. route (Harvey *et al.*, 1975) but the oral form is not suitable for long-term control of seizures. The half-life is only 46 min. Chlormethiazole is relatively free from cardiorespiratory depressant effects. It is formulated for i.v. infusion as 4 g in 500 ml given over 6–8 h, adjusted according to the patient's response. It may also be given as bolus injections of 1.2–3 g i.v., but this is less satisfactory than infusions in view of the short half-life.

UNCOMMONLY USED ANTICONVULSANTS

There are a number of drugs which are now seldom used because they have been superseded by more effective or less toxic alternatives. They are briefly mentioned below because some patients may still be maintained on them but they are not recommended for new therapy.

Sulthiame

This is a sulphonamide derivative with anticonvulsant effects in experimental seizures. Clinical trials have been unimpressive as early reports were based on poorly controlled studies in which sulthiame was given in combination with other drugs. Some of the anticonvulsant effects may have occurred because sulthiame inhibits the metabolism of phenytoin and barbiturates. Green *et al.* (1974) in a controlled trial found it of little value compared to phenytoin.

The usual dose is 200 mg t.i.d. in adults and children over the age of 6 years, and 100 mg t.i.d. for children of 1–5 years. It may result in sedation, hyperventilation, paraesthesiae in the extremities, anorexia and weight loss.

Trimethadione and paramethadione

These are of historical interest as early drugs which were selectively effective for petit mal but have proved to be both less effective and more toxic than ethosuximide and its newer rival sodium valproate.

Acetazolamide

Acetazolamide is a sulphonamide derivative which inhibits carbonic anhydrase. The recommended dose is 250 mg daily or b.d. As tolerance develops rapidly it has little value for long-term control in the epilepsies but may be tried, usually with limited success, in women with menstrual seizures, starting the drug about a week before the expected period.

THE SELECTION OF ANTICONVULSANTS

The problem now is the selection of the best anticonvulsant for particular clinical situations. The decision should be made on the basis of careful comparative trials but sometimes good evidence is not available.

1. Petit mal

Until recently ethosuximide was clearly the treatment of choice but sodium valproate and clonazepam are now alternatives. Large comparative studies have yet to be done. Where the patient has petit mal only, ethosuximide remains a satisfactory choice. If grand mal also occurs then sodium valproate or clonazepam will allow the patient to be treated with a single drug. Sodium valproate has the advantage over clonazepam that it seldom produces sedative side-effects.

2. Focal or major generalised seizures

The aim is to control the patient's epilepsy with a single drug without significant adverse effects. The main contenders for selection are the barbiturates, phenytoin, carbamazepine, sodium valproate and clonazepam. Generalised seizures are easier to prevent than focal ones, and in many patients a complete abolition of focal seizures cannot be achieved regardless of the anticonvulsant drug. The majority of patients presenting to a neurological clinic can be controlled on monotherapy. Many controlled trials have shown little differences in the effectiveness of the main anticonvulsants. No significant differences in seizure control were found in a trial of phenytoin, phenobarbitone and primidone (White *et al.*, 1966); carbamazepine, phenytoin and phenobarbitone (Cereghino *et al.*, 1974); carbamazepine and phenytoin (Troupin *et al.*, 1977); primidone and phenytoin in children (Millichap and Aymat, 1968). Phenytoin was thought to be slightly more effective than primidone (Cereghino *et al.*, 1974). Controlled trials of sodium valproate with longer-established anticonvulsants have not yet been performed, but it is likely that it will prove just as effective.

The choice is therefore not made on efficacy of anticonvulsants but on the severity and frequency of adverse effects, the availability of blood levels to assist control, and the costs of the drugs. Phenytoin has become more popular than barbiturates because it is less sedative. It is considerably less expensive than sodium valproate or carbamazepine. Both carbamazepine and sodium valproate are less sedative than phenytoin and they do not result in hursutism, acne, and facial coarsening. They may, therefore, be more acceptable, particularly for young women.

Drug failures

Before a drug is considered as a failure a serum level should be measured, if possible, to establish if poor compliance or rapid metabolism is the cause of the apparent drug failure. If treatment fails on one drug a single alternative should be introduced to an adequate dose before withdrawing the first drug. If seizures continue on monotherapy then combinations of anticonvulsants are to be used. There is little objective evidence on the best combinations. One study has reported that primidone is as effective as carbamazepine in combination with phenytoin. Primidone and phenytoin produced slightly more depression and impairment on psychometric testing, but fewer mild adverse effects (Rodin *et al.*, 1976). The only drug combination which is contraindicated is the use of primidone and phenobarbitone, as both are barbiturate derivatives.

In children with refractory seizures, particularly minor motor seizures and myoclonic attacks, a ketogenic diet should be tried. If the diet incorporates 60 per cent of the calorie requirements as medium-chain triglycerides, spread throughout the day, it is less unpleasant, with fewer adverse effects than previous regimes (Huttenlocher *et al.*, 1971).

3. Myoclonus

Myoclonus may arise from a variety of causes and is at times frustratingly refractory to treatment. The benzodiazepines are, in general, the most satisfactory drugs. Browne and Penry (1973), reviewing the evidence, concluded that nitrazepam was slightly superior to diazepam but more recently clonazepam has become the treatment of choice. Other major anticonvulsants including sodium valproate may also reduce myoclonus.

When the myoclonus is secondary to anoxic brain damage, the movements may be reduced or abolished by treatment with 5-hydroxytryptophan, a 5-HT precursor. Because 5-hydroxytryptophan is very expensive for continued use, tryptophan and a monoamine oxidase inhibitor may be tried.

4. Status epilepticus

This subject has been carefully reviewed by Duffy and Lombroso (1978).

(a) Major status epilepticus

The immediate priority in this medical emergency is a secure airway.

The second priority is to stop the seizures. The convulsions result in major neuronal metabolic changes and if these are prolonged and compounded by hypoxia, oedema, and electrolyte changes, permanent cerebral damage or death may occur. Comparative trials of the various drugs available have not been done. Diazepam or clonazepam are now the most widely used and are administered by i.v. bolus injections as discussed previously. Phenytoin i.v. may be effective and it has the advantage that treatment may be continued after control of the status epilepticus. A loading regime is needed to achieve adequate plasma levels rapidly. Phenobarbitone i.m. is not suitable because of the delay in the onset of its action. Chlormethiazole i.v. is effective in some patients refractory to the benzodiazepines (Harvey *et al.*, 1975). Thiopentone i.v. may be effective (Brown and Horton, 1967) but it should be administered in an intensive care unit where ventilatory assistance is available. A dose of 25–100 mg by slow i.v. injection is recommended initially, then 1 g in 550 Ringer-lactate should be infused at a rate of 1 ml/min reducing to 0.5 ml/min in 30 min if the convulsions have ceased. Treatment may have to be continued for 48–72 h and assisted ventilation may be needed. If the patient is paralysed and ventilated then monitoring of the EEG paroxysmal activity is needed as the clinical features of the seizures are no longer apparent. A cerebral function monitor provides a simple continuous readout for this purpose. Paralysis and ventilation should be avoided unless there is effective monitoring of EEG activity.

Paraldehyde is effective and may still have a place in initial treatment at home by the family doctor, particularly if i.v. administration of drugs is not feasible, as in the infant. Because of the need for large-volume i.m. injections, the local tissue irritation and the impression that benzodiazepines or chlormethiazole are more effective it is now seldom used in hospital practice. If administered by a plastic syringe it must be drawn up immediately before it is given. Whitty and Taylor (1949) recommended 8–10 ml initially in adults. Further 5 ml doses may be given if the attacks have not ceased in 30 min. In children the dose is 0.15 mg/kg or 1 ml/year up to 10 years. Diazepam is an alternative to paraldehyde for i.m. administration.

Other measures for treatment of status epilepticus include the treatment of cerebral oedema with dexamethasone (10 mg i.v. or i.m. in adults or 0.1 mg/kg in children initially with a maintenance dose of 2–4 mg in adults or 0.05 mg/kg in children 6-hourly). Life-threatening cerebral oedema may be treated with mannitol using 300 ml of 20 per cent solution infused over 30 min. Hyperpyrexia is nursed with tepid sponging and cooling with a fan. Fluid and electrolyte disorders, and chest infections, should be treated.

(b) Petit mal status

Diazepam or clonazepam are the drugs of choice.

(c) Focal status epilepticus

Temporal lobe status or epilepsia partialis continua require a similar regime to that used for grand mal status although the need is not as urgent.

5. Febrile convulsions

This is a common problem confronting the family practitioner and the decisions in management may be considered for each of three situations which may arise.

(a) The single brief convulsion

The aim is to prevent further attacks during the fever by treating the infection, if possible, and reducing the temperature. If there is any suggestion of meningitis, if further observation at home would be un-reliable, or parents are very anxious, admission to hospital is indicated. The temperature should be reduced with tepid sponging, and aspirin or paracetamol. Phenobarbitone will not achieve an adequate serum level for at least 48 h, and is not indicated in this situation.

(b) Prolonged seizures

Attacks lasting longer than 30 min may be associated with brain damage, either mental retardation and/or subsequent epilepsy. Shorter seizures of 15–30 min may also carry such a risk but the evidence is less clear. A continuing seizure should be treated with i.v. diazepam or clonazepam as for status epilepticus. If i.v. administration is not feasible then i.m. diazepam or paraldehyde should be given. The pyrexia and underlying infection should be treated. Admission to hospital is preferable so that further convulsions may be treated promptly.

(c) Prevention of recurrent febrile convulsions

The risk of febrile convulsions in subsequent fevers is greater where the initial attack was in a younger patient of less than 19 months, with previous prolonged or recurrent seizures, a positive family history or a persistent neurological deficit. The EEG is not usually helpful in establishing a prognosis. The parents should be made aware of the need to recognise fever and to reduce the temperature. For prophylaxis, the choice now lies between phenobarbitone and sodium valproate. Phenobarbitone has been used more extensively and a daily dose of 3—4 mg/kg reduces significantly the risk of further convulsions if a plasma level is greater than 15 μg/ml (60 μmol/l) (Faero *et al.*, 1972). The main problem with this treatment is that about 20 per cent of children become over-active and irritable. Others fail to comply. The phenobarbitone should be gradually withdrawn at the age of 5 years and the child should not be labelled as epileptic at school. The treatment does not impair intellectual ability on subsequent testing. The alternative to phenobarbitone is sodium valproate which does not produce the hyperactivity but is more liable to cause nausea or diarrhoea (Wallace and Aldridge-Smith, 1980).

6. Pregnancy

A number of problems occur in pregnancy and are well reviewed by Montouris *et al.* (1979). Several studies report that the risk of malformation in patients on anticonvulsants is increased to two or three times the expected rate in the general population. Cleft lip and palate, and congenital heart disease, are the commonest abnormalities but others occur. In addition a fetal-hydantoin syndrome has been described (Hanson and Smith, 1975). A trimethadione syndrome is avoided by not using the drug. Carbamazepine and sodium valproate have not been used widely enough for the risks of teratogenic effects to be known. As the risks of having uncontrolled seizures during and after pregnancy appear greater than the small teratogenic risk, patients should remain on anticonvulsant therapy.

The metabolism of anticonvulsant drugs is altered during pregnancy. As the clearance of phenytoin and barbiturates is increased the serum levels tend to fall progressively and the dosage requirements increase. The metabolism reverts to normal in the early weeks after delivery. Therefore regular monthly serum level monitoring is useful during pregnancy, and the monitoring should be continued in the early weeks after delivery. The risk of seizures is increased during pregnancy but this finding may arise in part from the declining blood levels.

Phenobarbitone readily enters the breast milk and may contribute to neonatal drowsiness but phenytoin has not been implicated in this effect. Sodium valproate also enters breast milk but its effects on the neonate are not known.

An additional complication is that the production and release of vitamin K-dependent clotting factors may be depressed by phenytoin and phenobarbitone, causing neonatal bleeding.

7. Prophylaxis of post-traumatic epilepsy

The value of prophylactic therapy for patients with a high risk of developing post-traumatic epilepsy is uncertain. The risks of having late (after the first week) post-traumatic epilepsy is particularly high in patients with acute haematoma (31 per cent), early epilepsy (25 per cent) and depressed fractures (15 per cent) (Jennett, 1975). Late epilepsy develops more than 4 years after the injury in about 20 per cent of patients who develop epilepsy, and in these patients the frequency of seizures is greater and remission less likely than in patients developing the seizures earlier. Both focal and generalised seizures occur.

Phenytoin has not been shown to be valuable but further evidence is awaited. There is limited evidence that sodium valproate may be useful.

SURGERY

Surgical treatment can be effective in selected patients whose seizures are not controlled by adequate medication. Patients being considered for surgery need careful assessment in specialist units and the subject needs only brief discussion here.

Focal seizures

Abnormal tissues such as glial scars, small haematomas, etc. may cause focal seizures. The commonest site is the temporal lobe. These abnormalities are excised at operation, and although this inevitably leaves a scar the liability to seizures is diminished. Surgery should be considered in patients refractory to anticonvulsant therapy who have lateralised or predominantly lateralised EEG abnormalities. Good results are reported in children as well as adults, and in one series 50—60 per cent of patients were reported to become fit-free, with a lesser improvement in the remainder (Falconer, 1974). The surgery may improve disturbed behaviour as well as seizure control, and both the morbidity and the mortality are low. Usually tissue containing the focal abnormality is excised, but a different approach — lobotomy — has been used in which, under stereotactic control, tracts from the uncus, hippocampus and temporal lobe isthmus are sectioned.

Hemispherectomy

This radical procedure of massive hemidecortication has been used with surprising success in children with infantile hemiplegia, intractable epilepsy, behaviour disorder and mental retardation. Improvement of epilepsy, behaviour and intellectual function has been reported but delayed onset of intracranial haemorrhage mars these results.

Corpus callosum section

This procedure has yielded a wealth of information on the functions of right and left hemispheres, but the success in control of seizures has been too modest for widespread use in the control of epilepsy arising from diffuse unilateral lesions.

Stereotactic lesions; subcortical and amygdala

Several small series of patients, with lesions at varying sites, have reported mixed success. Lesions have been made in subcortical systems involved in the production or propagation of discharges in the pallidum, fornix, field of Forel, ventroanterior nucleus or centromedianum nucleus of the thalamus. Destructive lesions in the amygdala have also been performed in patients with both behavioural problems and epilepsy, with greater success reported for behavioural problems than for epilepsy. There have been conflicting reports on whether temporal lobe or grand mal seizures are suppressed to a greater extent.

Chronic cerebellar stimulation

The considerable experimental evidence suggesting cerebellar involvement in the control of seizures led to the implantation of cerebellar electrodes for chronic stimulation. After the initial success subsequent reports have not been as satisfactory, and the technique is still under evaluation.

DISORDERS OF SLEEP

The development of sleep laboratories has produced more accurate classifications of disorders of sleep and arousal and the beginning of an understanding of their mechanisms. Although some disorders cannot be effectively treated it is helpful to recognise the nature of the problem.

Primary sleep disorders

Narcolepsy—cataplexy

The severity of cataplexy, the sudden involuntary weakening that occurs on an emotional reaction, must be assessed separately from narcolepsy, the irresistible, inappropriate desire for sleep. The other components of the syndrome, sleep paralysis and hypnogogic hallucinations, are less common. The syndrome can be regarded as a failure of synchronisation of normal mechanism of consciousness, sleep, and maintenance of muscle tone.

The sleep of narcolepsy may be dangerous — e.g. when driving — or embarrassing, although usually brief and refreshing. It may be treated with *d*-amphetamine usually 10 mg b.d. or t.i.d. and dependence is rare. Because of legal restrictions and anxiety about amphetamine abuse the alternative drug, methylphenidate, is usually preferable. It is given as 10 mg b.d. or t.i.d., avoiding giving it later than about 5 p.m. lest it interfere with night-time sleep.

Cataplexy is mild in some patients, and if they can avoid emotional precipitants drug therapy is not required. Tricyclic drugs are used in the more severely affected patients and clomipramine is the treatment of choice. This drug has more marked effects on 5-HT re-uptake than on noradrenaline and dopamine. The dose is 25 mg nocte, with gradual increments every 1—2 weeks to 75—100 mg daily. It may for convenience be given as a single night-time dose. If the patient is intolerant of 25 mg then a 10 mg dose should be given and the increments made more slowly. The possible adverse effects are those of the tricyclic group — anticholinergic effects, postural hypotension, cardiac arrhythmias, tremor, ataxia, anxiety, agitation, drowsiness, confusion, and occasional reports of seizures. Clomipramine sometimes improves sleep paralysis and hypnogogic hallucinations.

Sleep apnoea

This is an important cause of excessive day-time sleepiness. The diagnosis is suggested if the patient snores excessively and has periods of apnoea. Laboratory observations have shown these to be accompanied by intense cyanosis and hypertension. One form of sleep apnoea arises from a failure of central drive to respiration of unknown cause. Treatment is generally ineffective although tricyclic drugs have been reported to help occasionally. The alternative mechanism for apnoea during sleep is airways obstruction from collapse of the upper respiratory tract. The obstruction may be mechanical in the larynx, the soft palate, or associated with an abnormal jaw, or it may be secondary to a central lesion. Severely affected patients may be helped with a tracheostomy with a valve which can be opened in the night and closed by day.

There are a number of rare primary sleep disorders mainly diagnosed in the sleep laboratory. In *nocturnal myoclonus* sleep is disturbed by severe myoclonus and is to be distinguished from the common jerking on falling asleep, and also from the 'restless legs' syndrome. Benzodiazepines reduce the severity of the myoclonus. In *non-restorative sleep* runs of alpha rhythms intrude periodically into sleep, and tricyclic drugs occasionally help. In the related disorder of *neutral state* syndrome runs of 'microsleeps' occur in the day and 'micrawakes' during sleep. Treatment is ineffective. In another disorder sleep is interrupted by awakenings from REM sleep, and chlordiazepoxide may help. The *Kleine—Levin syndrome* may be helped with methylphenidate or amphetamine. In the remarkable syndrome of *periodic hypersomnia* prolonged periods of sleep lasting for days occurs at intervals of several weeks, months or even 2 years. Treatment is unsatisfactory.

Secondary sleep disorders

Medical causes of excessive day-time sleepiness and disturbed sleep are usually easily distinguished from the primary sleep disorders. These include various neurological disorders affecting the hypothalamus, epilepsy, chronic pain, hypnotic abuse and taking an excess of stimulants such as coffee. Psychiatric disorders are more difficult to assess and the treatment is that of the underlying depression, anxiety state, alcoholism, or behaviour disorder.

Parasomnias

Sleepwalking occurs more commonly in children than in adults, is usually not the result of psychological stress, and does not occur during dreaming. It is potentially dangerous in some situations, e.g. in a high flat where a subject may step through a window. In the persistent sleepwalker in dangerous situations it is wise to lock doors and attempt to reduce the danger. Diazepam or tricyclic drugs are not reliably effective. *Night terrors* occur during slow-wave sleep and *nightmares* during the dream activity associated with REM sleep. Both *bruxism,* the grinding of the teeth during sleep, and violent *jerking head movements* (jactio capitis nocturna) disturb relatives more than patients. Treatment is unsatisfactory and is restricted to attempts to reduce injury.

REFERENCES

Aarli, J A (1976) Drug-induced IgA deficiency in epileptic patients. *Archives of Neurology*, 33, 291—299.

Brown, A S and Horton, J M (1967) Status epilepticus treated by intravenous infusions of thiopentone sodium. *British Medical Journal*, 1, 27—28.

Browne, T R and Penry, J K (1973) Benzodiazepines in the treatment of epilepsy. *Epilepsia*, 14, 277—310.

Bruni, J and Wilder, B J (1979) Valproic acid. Review of a new anti-epileptic drug. *Archives of Neurology*, 36, 393—398.

Bureau, M, Guey, J, Dravet, C and Roger, J (1968) A study of the distribution of petit mal absences in the child in relation to his activities. *ECG and Clinical Neurophysiology*, 25, 513.

Cereghino, J J, Brock, J T, Van Meter, J C, Penry, J K, Smith, L D and White, B G (1974) Carbamazepine for epilepsy. A controlled prospective evaluation. *Neurology*, 24, 401—410.

Duffy, F H and Lombroso, C T (1978) *Treatment of Status Epilepticus. Clinical Neuropharmacology*, Vol. 3 (Ed) H L Klawans. Raven Press, New York.

Faero, O, Kastrup, K W, Lykkegaard-Nielsen, E, Melchior, J C and Thorn, I (1972) Successful prophylaxis of febrile convulsions with phenobarbital. *Epilepsia*, 13, 279—285.

Falconer, M A (1974) Mesial temporal (Ammon's horn) sclerosis as a common cause of epilepsy. *Lancet*, 2, 767—771.

Forster, F M (1972) The classification and conditioning treatment of the reflex epilepsies. *International Journal of Neurology*, 9, 73—86.

Friis, M L and Lund, M (1974) Stress convulsions. *Archives of Neurology*, 31, 155—159.

Green, J R, Troupin, A S, Helpern, L M, Friel, P and Kanarek, P (1974) Sulthiame: evaluation as an anticonvulsant. *Epilepsia*, 15, 329.

Hanson, J W and Smith, D W (1975) The fetal hydantoin syndrome. *Journal of Paediatrics*, 87, 285—290.

Harvey, P K P, Higgenbottam, T W and Loh, L (1975) Chlormethiazole in treatment of status epilepticus. *British Medical Journal*, 2, 603—605.

Huttenlocher, P R, Wilbourn, A J and Signore, J M (1971) Medium-chain triglycerides as a therapy for intractable childhood epilepsy. *Neurology*, 21, 1097—1103.

Jennett, B (1975) *Epilepsy after Non-missile Head Injuries.* Heinemann, London.

Johnson, L C, De Bolt, W L, Long, M T, Ross, J J, Sassin, J F, Arthur, R J and Walter, R D (1972) Diagnostic factors in adult males following initial seizures. *Archives of Neurology*, 27, 193—197.

Laks, S and Korczyn, A D (1977) Epilepsy and driving in Israel. In: *Epilepsy. The Eighth International Symposium*, pp. 307—311. (Ed) J K Penry. Raven Press, New York.

Lindsay, J, Ounsted, C and Richards, P (1979) Long-term outcome in children with temporal lobe seizures. I. Social outcome and childhood factors. *Developmental Medicine and Child Neurology*, 21, 285—298.

Livingstone, S and Berman, W (1973) Participation of epileptic patients in sports. *Journal of the American Medical Association*, **224**, 236–238.

Millichap, J C and Aymat, F (1968) Controlled evaluation of primidone and diphenylhydantoin sodium. Comparative anticonvulsant efficacy and toxicity in children. *Journal of the American Medical Association*, **204**, 738–739.

Montouris, G D, Fenichel, G M and McLain, L W (1979) The pregnant epileptic. A review and recommendation. *Archives of Neurology*, **36**, 601–603.

Mostofsky, D I (1977) Behaviour therapy for seizure control. In: *Epilepsy. The Eighth International Symposium*, pp. 239–243. (Ed) J K Perry. Raven Press, New York.

Pampiglione, G and Da Costa, A A (1975) Intravenous therapy and EEG monitoring in prolonged seizures. *Journal of Neurology, Neurosurgery and Psychiatry*, **38**, 371–377.

Perucca, Ed, Garratt, A, Hebdige, S and Richens, A (1978) Water intoxication in epileptic patients receiving carbamazepine. *Journal of Neurology, Neurosurgery and Psychiatry*, **41**, 713–718.

Record, K E, Rapp, R P, Young, A B and Kostenbauder, H B (1979) Oral phenytoin loading in adults: rapid achievement of therapeutic plasma levels. *Annals of Neurology*, **5**, 268–270.

Reynolds, E H (1973) Anticonvulsants, folic acid and epilepsy. *Lancet*, **1**, 1376–1377.

Richens, A (1976) Clinical pharmacology and medical treatment. In: *A Textbook of Epilepsy*, p. 196. (Ed) J Laidlaw and A Richens. Churchill-Livingstone, Edinburgh.

Richens, A and Dunlop, A (1975) Serum phenytoin levels in management of epilepsy. *Lancet*, **2**, 247–248.

Rodin, E A (1968) *The Prognosis of Patients with Epilepsy*. C C Thomas, Springfield, Illinois.

Rodin, E A, Rim, C S, Kitano, H, Lewis, R and Rennick, P M (1976) A comparison of the effectiveness of primidone versus carbamazepine in epileptic out patients. *Journal of Nervous and Mental Disorders*, **163**, 41–46.

Rowan, A J, Binnie, C D, Warfield, C A, Meinardi, H and Meijer, J W (1979) The delayed effect of sodium valproate on the photoconvulsive response in man. *Epilepsia*, **20**, 61–68.

The Royal Commission on Accident Prevention (1976) *Medical Aspects of Fitness to Drive*. (Ed) A Raffle.

Sommerbeck, K W, Theilgaard, A, Rasmussen, K E, Løhren, V, Gram, L and Wulff, K (1977) Valproate sodium: evaluation of so-called psychotropic effect. A controlled study. *Epilepsia*, **18**, 157–159.

Trimble, M R and Reynolds, E H (1976) Anticonvulsant drugs and mental symptoms: a review. *Psychological Medicine*, **6**, 169–178.

Troupin, A S, Ojemann, L M, Halpern, L, Dodrill, C, Wilkus, R, Friel, P and Feigl, P (1977) Carbamazepine — a double-blind comparison with phenytoin. *Neurology*, **27**, 511–519.

Vajda, F J E, Mihaly, G W and Miles, J L (1978) Rectal administration of sodium valproate in status epilepticus. *Neurology*, **28**, 897–899.

Wallace, S J and Aldridge-Smith, J (1980) Successful prophylaxis against febrile convulsions with valproic acid or phenobarbitone. *British Medical Journal*, **280**, 353–354.

White, P T, Plott, D and Norton, J (1966) Relative anticonvulsant potency of primidone. A double-blind comparison. *Archives of Neurology*, **14**, 31–35.

Whitty, C W M and Taylor, M (1949) Treatment of status epilepticus. *Lancet*, **2**, 591.

Wilder, B J, Serrano, E E, Ramsey, E and Buchanan, R A (1974) A method for shifting from oral to intramuscular diphenylhydantoin administration. *Clinical Pharmacology and Therapeutics*, **16**, 507–513.

Wulff, K, Flachs, H, Wurtz-Jorgensen, A (1977) Clinical pharmacological aspects of sodium valproate. *Epilepsia*, **18**, 149–157.

CHAPTER THREE

Cerebrovascular Disease

PREVENTION OF STROKE

Although there have been exciting advances in the study of atherogenesis, and in platelet function, these have not yet resulted in major
developments in the prevention of strokes. The main aim in stroke prevention is to recognise and treat the small proportion of patients with
diseases other than atheroma, and to treat both transient ischaemic
attacks and hypertension.

1. Transient ischaemic attacks (TIA)

TIAs are arbitrarily defined as episodes of transient neurological dysfunction, presumed to be ischaemic in origin, lasting less than 24 h. The
management problems are similar in patients with small strokes that
recover completely in more than 24 h (reversible ischaemic neurological
deficits) and those with only minimal residual dysfunction after a major
ischaemic attack. TIAs must be distinguished from other transient disorders such as focal epilepsy, migraine, and Meniere's syndrome. The
aim of treatment is to prevent further TIAs and stroke. The risk of
developing a stroke in a patient with TIAs has been variously reported.
Some of the larger series find the risk of having a stroke within 5 years
to be 30–40 per cent for the attacks arising in the carotid distribution,
and lower risks for those in the vertebrobasilar artery distribution. The
greatest risk is in the first year after the onset of TIAs, and over 50 per
cent of patients will have ceased having further TIAs at 3 years.

In many patients the ischaemic attacks arise from platelet emboli
from the heart or from atheromatous plaques in the extracranial vessels.
Emboli from the carotid bifurcation are particularly important as they
are accessible for surgery. Some attacks may arise from a haemodynamic
crisis when there is transient reduction in cerebral perfusion, e.g. during
cardiac arrhythmias, or when compression of the vertebral artery or

kinking of the carotid artery occurs during neck movement. The older idea of cerebral arterial 'spasm', as a cause of TIA is impossible to confirm or refute.

Assessment of patients with TIA

Clinical assessment should include examination of erect and supine BP, the heart, the neck vessels for bruits, the optic fundus for the retinopathy of hypertension or other vascular diseases and tenderness of temporal and occipital arteries. Non-atheromatous disorders must be considered because their treatment is different. Patients should have a haemoglobin and haematocrit for anaemia or polycythaemia. A VDRL test, ESR, and possibly ANF should be done in the search for a vasculitis such as meningovascular syphilis, cranial arteritis, or polyarteritis nodosa. If a connective tissue disorder is present, macroglobulinaemia should be considered because this may result in high viscosity and poor cerebral perfusion. If there is a history of palpitations or if the attacks consist of dizziness, faintness, darkness of vision or blackouts, then 24 h ambulatory ECG monitoring may reveal important dysrhythmias. Minor, infrequent dysrhythmias are difficult to interpret because they are common in the general population. An ECG may show evidence of recent myocardial infarction, a possible source of embolism. Rheumatic or other forms of heart disease may be carefully assessed. The EEG may be normal after a TIA. A focal abnormality may be present after a persistent ischaemic lesion or another pathology such as tumour. Paroxysmal features may suggest that the attacks were focal seizures. A CT scan is usually unnecessary in the patient with hypertension, bruits, and a history that is very clearly that of TIA, but is helpful in patients without such clear clinical features as a tumour may occasionally present with transient symptoms.

Transient monocular impairment of vision from retinal ischaemia (amaurosis fugax) is to be distinguished from early glaucoma and papilloedema and managed in a similar manner to other forms of TIA.

Treatment

Non-atheromatous disease should be treated appropriately (*see* separate sections for arteritis, meningovascular syphilis). It is very important that hypertension should be treated effectively. Most patients with TIAs have no evidence of vasculitis, hyperviscosity, serious cardiac arrhythmias or an expanding intracranial lesion. Their treatment is based on the concept that the TIAs arise from thromboembolism and the treatments available are surgery, anticoagulation and drugs which act on platelets.

Surgery

In carotid endarterectomy atheromatous plaques are removed, usually at the carotid bifurcation. Mild and moderate stenosis are commonly sources of platelet or cholesterol emboli but flow through stenosed vessels is reduced only if the narrowing is greater than 80 per cent. Surgical techniques have improved in recent years and in good centres the complication rate is low, less than 2 per cent (Thompson, 1979a). The recurrence rate of TIA after surgery is surprisingly low. The risks of surgery are greater if bilateral carotid arterial disease is present as both sides may require surgery. Vertebral angiography gives a more complete study but is not essential as few centres are prepared to correct abnormalities of the vertebral arteries. Where medical centres do not have expertise in vascular surgery the high risks eliminate endarterectomy as a realistic choice.

An interesting new surgical approach is the anastomosis of the superficial temporal artery to a branch of the middle cerebral artery in patients with carotid occlusion or intracranial arterial stenosis. The mortality and morbidity are low and after the anastomosis there is gradual increase in flow in subsequent months (Zumstein *et al.*, 1979). The procedure is still under evaluation. An occluded carotid artery is not suitable for direct surgery.

The physician's problem is the selection of patients for angiography and referral for surgery. The very frail, and patients with other major disease, should not be considered. The majority of patients will be over the age of 65, but age is not, in itself, a bar to surgery. A carotid bruit is a good indication of carotid arterial disease, but its absence does not preclude atheromatous narrowing at the carotid bifurcation. Direct low puncture of the common carotid artery or retrograde aortic catheterisation with selective cannulation of the carotid and/or vertebral arteries should show the extracranial vessels and the major intracranial arteries. The choice of technique depends on the expertise and preference of the radiologist. About half the patients with carotid distribution TIAs have stenosis or occlusion (Pessin *et al.*, 1977). Non-invasive techniques such as oculoplethysmography and ultrasound techniques are being developed. They may detect severe stenosis or occlusion but are still unreliable for the detection of mild and moderate degrees of stenosis from which emboli may arise. Therefore angiography remains essential for patients being considered for surgery.

Anticoagulation

Despite numerous studies the place of anticoagulation has not been established. In a critical review Brust (1977) draws attention to the poor design of most studies. Although there is some evidence for the value of anticoagulants, he concludes that the hypothesis that anti-coagulants may be of benefit in TIA is unproven. As the risk of stroke is greatest in the early months after the onset of TIA (Whisnant *et al.*, 1973), it is reasonable to suggest that if anticoagulants are to be given at all, they should be given for an initial 3—6-month period. Warfarin is the anticoagulant of choice. It inhibits vitamin K-dependent coagulation Factors II, VII, IX and X. Platelet aggregation is only indirectly affected, secondary to changes in thrombin. The dose range is 3—30 mg daily under regular laboratory control. Bleeding, including cerebral haemorrhage, is the most serious complication and vitamin K reverses its effect. As the half-life is 42 h, and the half-life of the coagulation factors varies between 6 and 60 h, a plateau in its effects does not occur for about a week. The drug interactions with its plasma binding or hepatic metabolism are extensive, and discussed in standard therapeutic texts.

Drugs acting on platelets

As platelet adhesion and aggregation are reduced with aspirin, dipyr-amidol or sulphinpyrazone these drugs have been used in the attempt to prevent platelet thromboembolism. There have been two major studies of aspirin in the treatment of TIAs. Fields *et al.* (1977) reported modest benefits from aspirin in a careful double-blind multicentre trial of aspirin 650 mg b.d. against a placebo in patients with carotid distri-bution TIAs. Significantly better results with aspirin therapy than placebo were found only when the prevention of further TIA, subse-quent stroke and death were considered together, but not when each of the end-points were considered independently. Better results were found in patients with multiple TIAs than after a single attack, and in patients with carotid lesions demonstrated at angiography. A larger study (Canadian Co-operative Study Group, 1978) found that aspirin 325 mg q.i.d. reduced the risk of death or stroke by 48 per cent in men, but the reduction by only 10 per cent in women was not statistically significant. There was no benefit from sulphinpyrazone.

The optimal dose of aspirin is not known, for there are two conflict-ing effects. Aspirin irreversibly inhibits cyclo-oxygenase, a platelet enzyme that produces the powerful pro-aggregatory substance throm-boxane A_2. But it also reversibly inhibits in the vessel wall the produc-

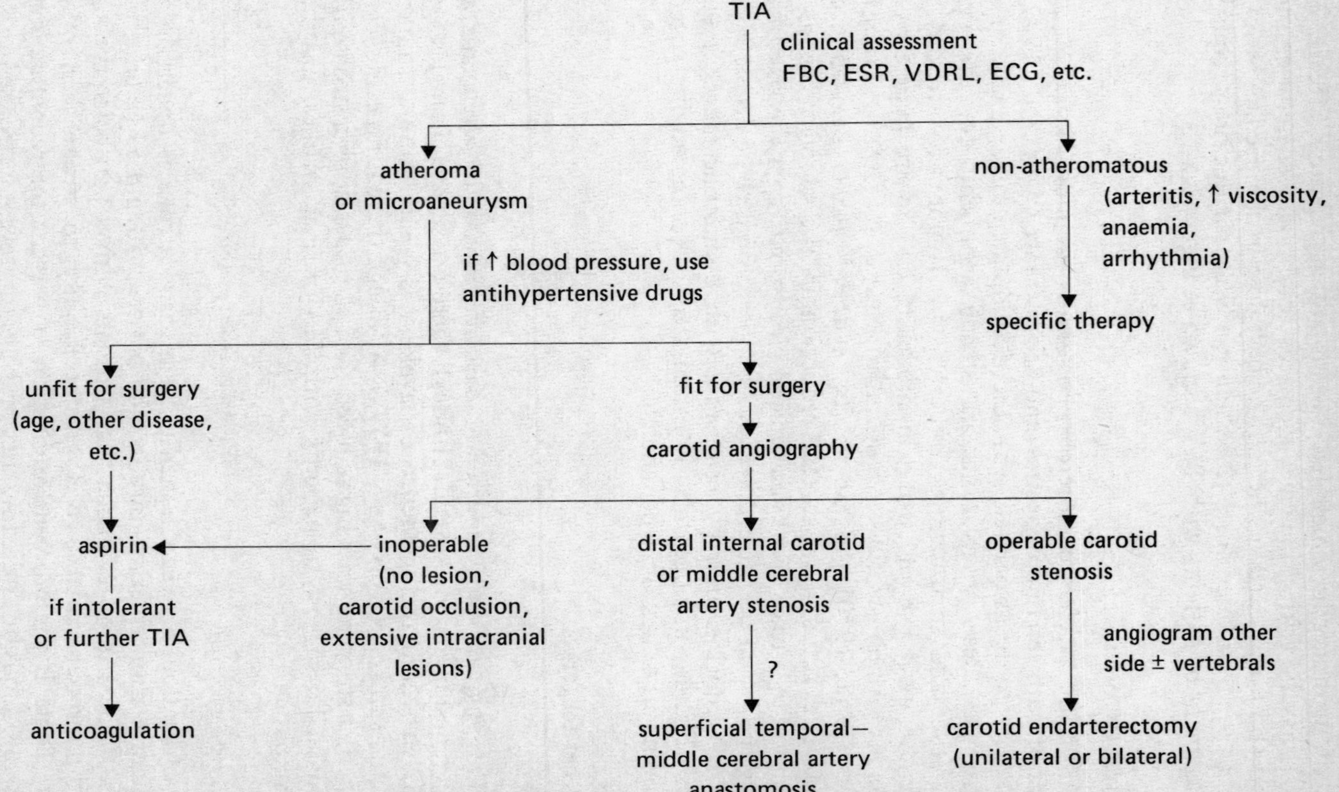

Figure 3.1   Decisions in the management of TIA

tion of prostacyclin which has potent anti-aggregatory effects. The
dosage may be critical in achieving a satisfactory balance between these
effects and it is uncertain whether the best dose is that used in the major
trials or much smaller doses. A scheme showing the decisions requiring
management of patients with TIA is shown in Figure 3.1.

2. Hypertension

Hypertension accelerates atherogenesis and is the most important precursor of both cerebral infarction and haemorrhage (Wolf *et al.*, 1977a).
It is particularly associated with the development of cerebral microaneurysms. These observations are strong arguments for the early
recognition and treatment of hypertension. Hypotensive therapy reduces the incidence of stroke in moderate and severe hypertension
(Veterans Administration Co-operative Study on Antihypertensive
Agents, 1967, 1970) and the risk of recurrent stroke (Beevers *et al.*,
1973). The benefits of careful reduction in the blood pressure of
patients with stroke and hypertension clearly outweigh the risk of reducing the blood pressure. Excessive hypotension is to be avoided. The
value of reducing mild hypertension, with a diastolic range of 90—
105 mmHg, has not been clearly established, but some studies suggest
that even this reduction is beneficial.

3. Other factors

Smoking

The Framingham study reported no clear relationship between smoking
and cerebral infarction overall, although there was a trend in males aged
50—59 in whom the incidence of stroke was greater among smokers
than non-smokers (Wolf *et al.*, 1977a). Although there is no evidence as
to whether stopping smoking reduced the risk of developing stroke, it is
reasonable to suggest to patients with TIA or small strokes that they
stop smoking.

Blood lipids

The association between hyperlipidaemia and stroke is uncertain. A
weak correlation emerges only in men between 50 and 59 (Wolf *et al.*,
1977a). There is no evidence that patients with a particular type of
hyperlipoproteinaemia have a greater liability to stroke than other
types. There is therefore no indication at present for recommending
that serum lipids be altered by diet or drugs to prevent a stroke.

Blood viscosity

The role of increased viscosity in causing stroke or extending an acute stroke needs study. Cerebral blood flow is reduced to a variable extent when the haematocrit is increased only slightly in the range 0.46–0.53. The reduction in cerebral blood flow is, however, consistent and increasingly marked with further increases in the haematocrit (Thomas *et al.*, 1977). This change in viscosity may be associated with an increased risk of stroke and might account for the observation in the Framingham study that patients with haemoglobin concentrations at the higher end of the 'normal' range have a greater risk of stroke. These observations suggest two implications. If there is a clear increase in viscosity, as in polycythaemia, a reduction of the haematocrit may reduce the risk of stroke. Furthermore dehydration, with resulting haemo-concentration, as may occur in an intercurrent infection in an elderly patient, may increase the liability to stroke.

Atrial fibrillation

Patients in atrial fibrillation have an increased risk of stroke. Wolf *et al.* (1977b) found the risk in patients with rheumatic heart disease to be about 17 times greater than the general population, and that in patients with chronic atrial fibrillation from other causes the risk was increased about 5 times that in the general population. There is a need for good controlled trials of anticoagulation in these groups of patients.

Oral contraceptives

The risk of stroke when taking oral contraceptives is increased (Collaborative Group for the Study of Stroke in Young Women, 1975) but the absolute risk remains low. This risk is increased more if the patient smokes or is hypertensive. If women develop TIAs or prominent migrainous symptoms (visual or other), oral contraceptives should not be prescribed.

Asymptomatic carotid bruits

A carotid bruit may be found during a routine medical assessment, or in the evaluation of patients with known ischaemic heart disease or peripheral vascular disease. The risk of developing TIAs or stroke is increased in these patients. Although a small number of surgeons with considerable expertise in carotid artery surgery operate on patients with asymptomatic carotid bruits (Thompson, 1979b), it is wise for most centres to be conservative lest the hazards outweigh the benefits. More commonly surgeons operate on the patients in two stages for bilateral carotid stenosis, first on the side on which emboli arise, then on the contralateral side.

Alcohol

A recent report on young men with strokes found that a high proportion occurred after bouts of heavy drinking (Hillbom and Keste, 1978). If further evidence confirms these observations it will be yet another argument against excessive alcohol consumption. The effect of moderate alcohol consumption on the risk of stroke is unclear.

THE ACUTE STROKE

Cerebral infarction arises either from cerebral arterial thrombosis or embolism. Cerebral haemorrhage may complicate microaneurysms, berry aneurysms, arterovenous malformations, established infarcts, or they may occur without clear cause. The management of a patient with stroke involves discussion of the prognosis, the decisions on how far to investigate the patient, the management of the acute stroke and the subsequent rehabilitation, if required.

Prognosis

Prediction of the prognosis at the time of presentation of an acute stroke is important for giving explanations to the patients and their relatives. Understanding the variable prognosis is also essential in assessing the value of reported treatments. About half the patients die in the first 3 weeks. The survival after cerebral haemorrhage is much poorer (16 per cent) than after infarction (84 per cent) (Marquardsen, 1969). The conscious level in the first 24 h, respiratory abnormalities, bilateral extensor plantar responses and conjugate gaze palsy indicate poor prognosis for survival. These observations are derived from the study of groups of patients, but it is difficult to be precise about the prognosis in an individual with stroke in the early stages. In the survivors of an acute stroke, a poor prognosis for satisfactory functional recovery is indicated by depressed consciousness and gaze palsy at the onset, and at 3 weeks by inability to walk unaided, a useless hand, and urinary incontinence (Matthews and Oxbury, 1975). Confusion, poor motivation and sensory defects also present major difficulties in rehabilitation.

Home versus hospital care

Some patients are satisfactorily managed at home. The family doctor may prefer this because a catastrophic illness requiring terminal care can be coped with at home, because of patients' and relatives' desires, a lack of hospital facilities, and the impression that hospital care adds little to the management of the patients. The arguments for hospital care are that it is easier to investigate patients, to provide nursing care in the acute phase, and to start rehabilitation. The value of an acute stroke unit has been doubted for some years. A recent controlled study found a lower morbidity in patients with moderately severe strokes treated in a stroke unit compared to general medical wards (Garraway *et al.*, 1980).

Investigation

The investigations should answer four questions that are important in the management of patients.

(1) Is there a non-atheromatous vascular disorder causing the stroke, such as cranial or syphilitic arteritis?

(2) Have systemic factors such as anaemia, polycythaemia or dehydration contributed to the stroke?

(3) Is there a cardiac cause either for embolism (rheumatic heart disease, recent myocardial infarction, subacute bacterial endocarditis) or has there been a cardiac arrhythmia?

(4) Is there an intracranial lesion suitable for surgical treatment, such as a berry aneurysm, a subdural or an intracerebral haematoma?

The investigations should therefore include a full blood count, ESR, VDRL, ECG, and chest X-ray. As a CT scan now permits recognition of abscess, intracranial haematomas, most tumours and hydrocephalus, it is an important non-invasive investigation for patients with an uncertain diagnosis. The increased X-ray absorption with haematoma is recognisable immediately after the stroke but the changes of infarction evolve gradually over the first 48 h; therefore haematomas which may require surgical treatment are readily differentiated from cerebral infarcts. Another value in recognising a haematoma is when considering anticoagulation to prevent a recurrent stroke — e.g. after cerebral embolism from rheumatic heart disease — for patients with a haematoma should not be anticoagulated. Unfortunately, even if an infarct is demonstrated on the CT scan, there is still a risk of secondary haemorrhage in the anticoagulated patient. Occasional subdural haematomas may be missed on the CT scan if they are isodense and bilateral. Isotope scanning (cerebral scintigraphy) may show changes after stroke but the information is much inferior to that produced by the CT scan.

Angiography

Angiography is indicated only if the management might be altered by making a clear diagnosis, e.g. in subdural haematoma, intracerebral haematoma, and meningioma.

Lumbar puncture

CSF examination is of limited value in the assessment of most patients with stroke. It is valuable if meningitis is a possibility or if the onset of the stroke was sudden, with headache and neck stiffness suggestive of subarachnoid haemorrhage. In patients with slowly evolving neck stiffness, a prodromal illness, cranial nerve palsies or positive blood serology, CSF may help in the search for meningovascular syphilis, tuberculous meningitis or other chronic encephalitides. The finding of xanthochromia in the CSF does not reliably differentiate cerebral haemorrhage from infarction. The problem is that blood may be found in the CSF when infarction is complicated by haemorrhage or it may be absent in a localised intracerebral haematoma. In most cases the management is not altered by distinguishing intracerebral haematoma from infarction.

EEG

The EEG seldom provides information of immediate value in management decisions. Prominent focal slow waves or, less commonly, spikes and sharp waves suggests a cortical lesion. In contrast, capsular damage produces less marked focal abnormality, although the hemiplegia or sensory defect may be severe. As cerebral haemorrhage does not usually involve the cortex primarily, it is less likely than infarction to produce major focal slow-wave abnormalities. Cerebral oedema with increased intracranial pressure and some brainstem lesions may be associated with bilateral EEG abnormalities.

Cerebral blood flow estimations

These are still research techniques although the development of intravenous and inhalation techniques has removed the need for direct puncture of the carotid arteries. Emission-tomographic scanning may be a reliable non-invasive method of studying cerebral perfusion in the future.

Management

Coma requires careful medical and nursing care (*see* Chapter 1). Additional medical conditions such as anaemia, cardiac failure, chest infection and dehydration must be treated.

Drug therapy

The results of drug treatment in acute stroke are disappointing. Many studies have been too late, with inadequate numbers, or poorly controlled. The broad aims of treatment have been to improve the microcirculation, reduce oedema, enhance defective neuronal metabolism and prevent the extension of thrombosis.

1. The microcirculation. Low molecular weight dextran has been used to reduce viscosity and prevent sludging and platelet aggregation in the ischaemic region. Intravenous dextran 40 in 5 per cent dextrose, 500 ml in the first hour, then 500 ml 12 hourly for 72 h reduced initial mortality, confirming previous studies, but follow-up at 6 months showed no difference between control and treated groups (Matthews *et al.*, 1976). Dextran combined with dexamethasone was no better than controls (Kaste *et al.*, 1976). Aminophylline has been reported to produce short-term improvement in some patients but not to influence the long-term recovery (Geismar *et al.*, 1976). Spasmolytic drugs such as isoproterenol and adrenergic blockers have not been fully assessed; 5 per cent CO_2 inhalation, a patent vasodilator, was ineffective in a controlled trial.

Hypertensive encephalopathy, now rare, requires urgent treatment to reduce the diastolic pressure to about 100—110 mmHg initially. In subsequent days the pressure can be reduced to lower levels, but excessive reductions are to be avoided. Sodium nitroprusside is administered *via* an infusion pump in a dosage range of 0.5—10 μg/kg per minute, but the rate is adjusted according to the hypotensive response. Alternatively diazoxide may be used but is liable to produce excessive fall in blood pressure unless it is used in small boluses of 100 mg, repeated every 5—10 min until the blood pressure has fallen sufficiently. Thereafter the hypotensive effect may be maintained by a β-blocker or hydrallazine, probably in combination with a diuretic.

Mild or moderate hypertension should not be treated in the acute phase. In many patients it declines spontaneously in the early days after the stroke. There are two problems with treatment of hypertension rapidly and soon after the stroke. Firstly, the autoregulatory range (the range of blood pressure over which blood flow is maintained constant) is increased above the normal range of mean pressure of 60–120 mmHg. Rapid reductions of blood pressure from the elevated hypertensive autoregulatory range results in disproportionate decreases in perfusion. The second problem is that the stroke itself impairs autoregulation and therefore treatment of the hypertension may produce disproportionate decrease in flow in the ischaemic region.

2. Cerebral oedema. Both cytotoxic and vasogenic oedema occur after acute stroke (pages 133–4). In cytotoxic oedema the anoxic intracellular damage results in cellular oedema with severe neuronal dysfunction. This form of oedema does not respond to steroids. In vasogenic oedema capillary permeability is defective and the resulting extracellular oedema is reduced by steroids. The balance of evidence from clinical studies is that dexamethasone does not improve the prognosis in patients with infarction, perhaps because cytotoxic oedema is dominant. A small group of patients with severe strokes and increased intracranial pressure might be improved but this requires study.

Gilsanz *et al.* (1975) found that i.v. glycerol, a dehydrating agent, produces significantly better results than dexamethasone, but the study only extended for 15 days. In a study with a longer follow-up no benefit was found (Larsson *et al.*, 1974).

3. Cerebral metabolism. A hopeful recent study in a double-blind controlled trial of naftidrofuryl (Praxilene) has been reported (Admani, 1978). This drug has an ill-defined protective action against the effects of cerebral ischaemia. Naftidrofuryl at 200 mg t.i.d. for 4 weeks, then 100 mg t.i.d. for 8 weeks, reduced the total disability score in a group of patients with recent stroke although the differences in each neurological function and in the activities of daily living were not great. Particularly important was the finding that the duration of stay in hospital was considerably shorter in the treated group. Further controlled studies are needed in which naftidrofuryl is started immediately after the onset of the stroke.

4. Anticoagulation. Anticoagulation is contraindicated in the acute stroke because of the risk of intracerebral haemorrhage. The only exception is the group of patients who slowly deteriorate and are labelled as having a progressing stroke or stroke-in-evolution. These patients require careful assessment for the slow deterioration may not arise from extension of the thrombosis but from cerebral oedema, haemorrhage, drug effects or metabolic abnormalities. Diagnosis of a progressing stroke is difficult because at the time of decision the deterioration may already be maximal. Nevertheless, studies in this group of patients suggest that anticoagulation improves the prognosis (Carter, 1961). Treatment should be with heparin initially then oral anticoagulants. Further studies are now needed using the CT scan which allows a more precise diagnosis. Patients with rheumatic heart disease and cerebral embolism should be anticoagulated but the best time for starting is unclear. Some physicians start immediately, others within a week, while some prefer to wait for 4 weeks because of the risk of secondary haemorrhage.

Surgery in the acute stroke

Emergency carotid endarterectomy for internal carotid artery occlusion has now been abandoned because of the disastrously high rate of haemorrhage. The value of surgical removal of intracerebral haematomata is uncertain. Dramatic improvement may occur in selected cases where there are 'mass' effects, i.e. evidence of shift of intracranial structures. However, follow-up of conservatively managed patients using a CT scan shows that even large haematomata are reabsorbed over several months. A benefit from surgery has yet to be shown in patients with intracerebral haematomata whose condition remains stable, without mass effects.

Subarachnoid haemorrhage

Ruptured intracranial aneurysm

The two major threats to the survivor of a ruptured berry aneurysm are rebleeding and the development of an ischaemic neurological deficit. The danger that haemorrhage may follow lysis of the thrombus at the point of previous rupture is greatest in the first 7–10 days. The risk diminishes thereafter but still persists as a risk of about 5 per cent per annum in subsequent years. Hypertension should be treated, if present. Technical and anaesthetic improvements have diminished the risks of surgery impressively in recent years but the timing of surgery remains difficult and vasospasm is not treated satisfactorily. Early surgery carries a greater risk of spasm and infarction with a lesser risk of rebleeding than a delayed operation. In recent years, antifibrinolytic drugs have been introduced to prevent the dissolution of the protective clot and thereby to delay or prevent a rebleeding. Epsilon-aminocaproic acid (EACA) was introduced first. It is given as an i.v. infusion of 30—36 g over 24 h or orally until surgery or for 6 weeks. Some studies have reported reduced mortality from rebleeding and others no clear difference. Tranexamic acid is a more potent antifibrinolytic drug and may result in stronger thrombi. It is of interest that in two patients having late direct surgery after tranexamic acid treatment dense adhesions around the aneurysm were found (Maurice-Williams, 1978). Both tranexamic acid and EACA carry a risk of inducing coagulation. Because of this risk of thrombosis the clot lysis time or fibrin degradation products should be monitored. Tranexamic acid reduces the risk of rebleeding in patients who do not proceed to surgery (Maurice-Williams, 1978). Although tranexamic acid appears useful in the treatment of patients unsuitable for operation, the treatment of choice in patients with little or no deficit is surgery. Further studies are needed to establish the place, if any, of antifibrinolytic drugs in this group of patients, balancing the risk of rebleeding against those of inducing cerebral thrombosis or more generalised thrombosis. Arteriovenous malformations may be excised if small, accessible and not in a critical area.

REHABILITATION

Rehabilitation of the stroke patient should start at the onset of the illness, taking into account the neurological deficits, the patients' previous personality, past illnesses and the domestic situation. An explanation of the problems such as dysphasia, hemianopia and sensory inattention should be given to the relatives or others caring for the patient. Several problems in rehabilitation need to be considered.

1. Dysphasia

Language defects must be distinguished from deafness, dementia, or confusional states. The assessment of language is a complex subject which cannot be discussed here. For most practical purposes the recognition of sensory, mixed and motor dysphasia is sufficient. Speech therapy techniques vary considerably and the value of each method has not been established. Clinical experience suggests that the severely affected patients — particularly with major receptive problems — make little progress, and that patients with mild dysphasias make adequate progress without speech therapy. A moderately affected patient provides the greatest scope for potential improvement. Recently enthusiastic, non-professional volunteers have been shown in preliminary studies to produce similar results in patients in the community to those obtained by trained speech therapists (Meikle *et al.*, 1979). The trained speech therapist is important in the hospital rehabilitation team, particularly in devising and assessing programmes of therapy. Material of appropriate complexity for practice in reading, writing and speaking is selected. Such material should be orientated to the patient's interests and be appropriate for his or her educational background. Many patients fatigue easily and sessions should be short, e.g. under 30 min. Comprehension is easier if the patient can see the speaker's facial expression, and if speech is slower and simpler than usual. Lay therapists are probably most useful in the community, stimulating, encouraging and supporting patients and their relatives.

2. Vision

Visual problems such as cataract or refractive error must be clearly distinguished from those arising from the stroke such as hemianopia, quadrantanopia, visual agnosia, and inattention. Any problems must be explained to the staff and relatives. The hemianopic patient should be approached from the side of intact vision and difficulties with reading, eating and walking should be appreciated. Both hemianopia and visual inattention are hazardous for driving, although the patient may adapt remarkably to hemianopia in other activities.

3. Intellectual impairment

A confusional state may arise from inappropriate drug therapy such as hypnotics or tranquillisers, or from treatable metabolic problems such as hypoxia or hyponatraemia. Such a toxic or metabolic confusional state should be distinguished from the usually transient drowsiness that may occur with an acute stroke, and from dysphasias. In addition, the presence of dementia is a serious bar to successful rehabilitation. Full psychometric assessment is unnecessary for the routine assessment of the patient with stroke. Nevertheless, assessment should be made of dysphasia, ability to perform mental arithmetic, orientation, recall of recent events, concentration or distractibility, mood and motivation, and the ability to conceptualise, for example, in the interpretation of proverbs. Sometimes the dementia is so gross that special evaluation is unnecessary. The more important groups are mildly affected patients with depression, anxiety or dysphasia complicating the assessment. In a busy ward with changing junior staff standardised testing is helpful (Isaacs, 1971).

4. Mood

Depression is common after a stroke and may be reduced by good overall care of the patient. It may, however, be an unrecognised cause of poor recovery after stroke and there is some evidence that tricyclic antidepressants help.

5. Anxiety

Both the patients and the family may be anxious. Employment, financial and domestic problems and the immediate incapacity are all considerable worries. Occasionally families may blame the stroke on psychological problems, e.g. worry or guilt, and an explanation of the nature of a stroke, its likely long-term effects, and the help which may be available is required for all patients and families.

6. Epilepsy

Either focal or generalised seizures may occur in about 6 per cent of patients after a stroke (Marquardsen, 1969). Therefore, the occurrence of seizures after a stroke is not an indication for extensive investigation for alternative diagnoses unless there are additional new clinical features. There are no comparative drug trials for the treatment of epilepsy in the elderly. Further attacks are usually prevented with phenytoin (Chapter 2).

7. Motor disorders

The motor problems in hemiparesis are complex. Weakness, spasticity, abnormal patterns of contraction and relaxation of muscles, and sensory function are important.

Passive movement

The early use of passive movement of the affected limbs is important to retain joint mobility, prevent contracture, and perhaps also to facilitate the return of voluntary function. This should be done by a physiotherapist, the nursing staff and/or family.

Posture

The limbs should be supported while sitting to avoid undue strain on soft tissues, particularly the shoulder. Subluxation at the shoulder may occur and is prevented by supporting the arm in a partially abducted position with slight elbow flexion, and by lifting the patient to avoid traction on the arm. Correct positioning prevents pressure palsies such as radial, ulnar and lateral popliteal palsy.

Spasticity

Mild or moderate spasticity may improve during physiotherapy but severe spasticity is difficult to treat. Baclofen may be used; if unsuccessful, dantrolene or diazepam are alternatives (Chapter 7). Unfortunately these drugs are disappointingly ineffective in the face of gross spasticity after a stroke. Cooling reduces spasticity temporarily. Intraneural and intramuscular motor point injections of phenol have been described for spasticity but have not come into widespread use. Intrathecal phenol, which reduces spasticity by damaging lumbar roots, is more valuable in patients with spinal cord lesions than in hemiparesis.

Contracture

The immobility of unrelieved spasticity may result in contracture. If this contracture is refractory to energetic physiotherapy and uncontrolled by an orthosis, it may be helped by section and transplantation of tendons. An equinovarus deformity may be corrected with elongation of the Achilles tendon combined with insertion of part of the tibialis anterior into the lateral border of the foot. Division of the flexors of the forearm may help major pronation—flexion deformities in the forearm and hand.

Physiotherapy

Different therapeutic approaches have been used in an attempt to correct the motor abnormalities in hemiparesis. They have not been compared in a controlled manner. One system encourages movement by allowing the basic synergistic contraction of limbs to develop, even if pathological, with the attempt to train or modify these movements subsequently. A contrasting approach argues that gross pathological synergistic flexion and extension movements should not be encouraged. Indeed they should be inhibited until there is enough recovery for selective movements to occur. Until superiority of one or a combination of techniques is shown the best results will come from a keen physiotherapist, systematically working with the patient using the techniques of motor control that he or she likes best. The physiotherapist should set goals and encourage hard work at rehabilitation. Training in balance, co-ordination, and walking, with or without an orthosis or Zimmer aid, should be given.

Orthoses

Unfortunately, orthotic devices are relatively ineffective with marked spasticity but are more useful in mild and moderately affected patients. Below-knee calipers and ankle-braces provide an established, ugly, robust device. The alternative polypropylene orthoses combine strength with lightness and are less obvious. Many hemiparetic patients learn to walk satisfactorily without the use of such a device.

Apraxias

Defective skilled movement in the absence of weakness, sensory impairment, extrapyramidal or cerebellar disorder arise from lesions of the parietal or frontal cortex. It is important to recognise their nature so that the patient is not misinterpreted as being demented, lacking in motivation or hysterical. Disorders of visio-spacial perception affect the rehabilitation profoundly, making tasks such as eating, dressing, getting into and out of bed, difficult.

Sensory loss

The striking problems of hemiparesis and spasticity usually overshadow the less obvious problems of sensory impairment but this sensory loss makes rehabilitation more difficult. In particular, sensory inattention is a profound handicap because the patient may neglect the affected side.

Aids to independence

The patient should aim to return home where possible. An increasing number of aids are now available and the patient's particular needs should be carefully and individually assessed. The access to the toilet, the provision of rails by the toilet or bath, non-slip mats in the bath, long-handled combs, thick-handled cutlery are all simple but important measures. If the patient is wheelchair-bound consideration of ramps, access to rooms, the type of wheelchair required, helping transfer to the toilet and to bed are all important. Electronic communication systems, such as the Possum, can be used to aid telephoning, opening doors, and controlling switches.

The support by the community

Each patient must again be assessed individually. In the United Kingdom the support may include 'meals-on-wheels', home help, visits from district nurses, attendance allowances, and day care. If support of the disabled patient at home is impossible then specially designed sheltered accommodation may be suitable. In the severely affected patient long-term institutional care is needed.

REFERENCES

Admani, A K (1978) New approach to treatment of recent stroke. *British Medical Journal*, **2**, 1678–1679.

Beevers, D G, Fairman, J E, Hamilton, M and Harpur, J E (1973) Antihypertensive treatment and the course of established cerebral vascular disease. *Lancet*, **1**, 1407–1409.

Brust, J C M (1977) Transient ischaemic attacks: natural history and anticoagulation. *Neurology*, **28**, 701–707.

Canadian Co-operative Study Group (1978) A randomised trial of aspirin and sulphinpyrazone in threatened stroke. *New England Journal of Medicine*, **299**, 53–59.

Carter, A B (1961) Anticoagulant treatment in progressing stroke. *British Medical Journal*, **2**, 70–73.

Collaborative Group for the Study of Stroke in Young Women (1975) Oral contraceptives and stroke in young women. Associated risk factors. *Journal of the American Medical Association*, **231**, 718–722.

Fields, W S, Lemak, N A, Frankowski, R F and Hardy, R J (1977) Controlled trial of aspirin in cerebral ischaemia. *Stroke*, **8**, 301–315.

Garraway, W M, Aktar, A J, Prescott, R J and Hockey, L (1980) Management of acute stroke in the elderly: preliminary results of a controlled trial. *British Medical Journal*, **1**, 1040–1043.

Geismar, P, Marquardsen, J and Sylvest, J (1976) Controlled trial of intravenous aminophylline in acute cerebral infarction. *Acta Neurologica Scandinavica*, **54**, 173–180.

Gilsanz, V, Rebollar, J L, Buencuerpo, J and Chantres, M T (1975) Controlled trial of glycerol versus dexamethasone in the treatment of acute cerebral infarction. *Lancet*, **1**, 1049–1051.

Hillbom, M and Kaste, M (1978) Does ethanol intoxication promote brain infarction in young adults? *Lancet*, **2**, 1181–1183.

Isaacs, B (1971) Identification of disability in the stroke patient. *Modern Geriatrics*, **1**, 390–401.

Kaste, M, Fogelholm, R and Waltimo, O (1976) Combined dexamethasone and low-molecular-weight dextran in acute brain infarction: double-blind study. *British Medical Journal*, **2**, 1409–1410.

Larsson, O, Marinovich, N and Barber, K (1974) Double-blind trial of glycerol therapy in early stroke. *Lancet*, **1**, 832–834.

Marquardsen, J (1969) The natural history of acute cerebrovascular disease: a retrospective study of 769 patients. *Acta Neurologica Scandinavica, Suppl.* 38.

Matthews, W B and Oxbury, J M (1975) Prognostic factors in stroke. In: *Outcome of Severe Damage to the Central Nervous System*, pp. 279—287. Ciba Symposium, Elsevier—Excerpta Medica—Holland.

Matthews, W B, Oxbury, J M, Grainger, K M R and Greenhall, R C D (1976) A blind controlled trial of dextran in the treatment of ischaemic stroke. *Brain,* **99,** 193—206.

Maurice-Williams, R S (1978) Prolonged antifibrinolysis: an effective non-surgical treatment for ruptured intracranial aneurysms? *British Medical Journal,* **1,** 945—947.

Meikle, M, Wechsler, E, Tupper, A, Berenson, M, Butler, J, Muthall, D and Stern, G (1979) Comparative trial of volunteer and professional treatment of dysphasia after stroke. *British Medical Journal,* **2,** 87—89.

Pessin, M S, Duncan, G W, Mohr, J P and Poskanzer, D C (1977) Clinical and angiographic features of carotid transient ischaemic attacks. *New England Journal of Medicine,* **296,** 358—362.

Thomas, D, Marshall, J, Ross-Russell, R W, Wetherley-Mein, G, Du Boulay, G H, Pearson, T C, Symon, L and Zilka, E (1977) Cerebral blood flow in polycythaemia. *Lancet,* **2,** 161—163.

Thompson, J E (1979a) Results of carotid surgery using an intraluminal shunt. In: *Progress in Stroke Research*, vol. 1. (Eds) R M Greenhalgh and F Clifford Rose. Pitman Medical, Tunbridge Wells.

Thompson, J E (1979b) The outcome of asymptomatic bruits. In: *Progress in Stroke Research*, vol. 1. (Eds) R M Greenhalgh and F Clifford Rose. Pitman Medical, Tunbridge Wells.

Veterans Administration Co-operative Study Group on Anti-hypertensive Agents (1967) Effects of treatment on morbidity in hypertension. *Journal of the American Medical Association,* **202,** 1028—1034.

Veterans Administration Co-operative Study Group on Anti-hypertensive Agents (1970) Effects of treatment on morbidity in hypertension. II. Results in patients with diastolic blood pressures averaging 90 through 114 mmHg. *Journal of the American Medical Association,* **213,** 1143—1152.

Whisnant, J P, Matsumoto, N and Elveback, L R (1973) The effect of anticoagulant therapy on the prognosis of patients with transient ischaemic attacks in a community. *Mayo Clinic Proceedings,* **48,** 844—848.

Wolf, P H, Dawber, T R, Thomas, H E and Kannel, W B (1977). Epidemiologic assessment of chronic atrial fibrillation and risk of stroke: the Framingham study. *Neurology,* **28,** 973—977.

Wolf, P A, Dawber, T R, Thomas, H E, Cotton, T and Kannel, W B (1977b) Epidemiology of stroke. *Advances in Neurology,* vol. 16, pp. 5—19. (Eds) R A Thompson and J R Green. Raven Press, New York.

Zumstein, B, Yasangil, M G and Yonekawa, Y (1979) Results of superficial temporal to middle cerebral artery bypass — review of 90 cases. *Progress in Stroke Research,* vol. 1. (Eds) R M Greenhalgh and F Clifford Rose. Pitman Medical, Tunbridge Wells.

CHAPTER FOUR

Parkinsonism

PATHOPHYSIOLOGICAL MECHANISMS

Although it has been appreciated since the early part of the century that Parkinson's disease is a disorder of the extrapyramidal system affecting particularly the substantia nigra, the nature of the underlying disturbance in terms of disordered physiology remains poorly understood. Early experimental studies on the basal ganglia in monkeys have shown that ablation of the caudate nucleus results in hyperactivity whereas stimulation brings about the arrest of spontaneous movement. Experimental lesions of the globus pallidus lead to a marked loss of postural reflexes. The basal ganglia are rich in both dopamine and acetylcholine and much of the dopamine present arises from cells in the substantia nigra whence it is carried along a dopaminergic pathway to be concentrated in the nerve terminals acting on the corpus striatum. A major outflow from the corpus striatum is via the globus pallidus and the ventrolateral nucleus of the thalamus and the effectiveness of surgical lesions in the globus pallidus or in the thalamus in relieving the tremor and rigidity of Parkinson's disease can perhaps be explained on the basis of these abnormal movements arising from a disordered function in this pathway and acting through the sensorimotor cortex. Studies of peripheral innervation in Parkinson's disease indicate that both alpha and gamma motor neurones are abnormally activated during Parkinsonian rigidity. Recordings from the ventrolateral nucleus in patients undergoing stereotactic surgery have also shown that neurones in this system fire at the tremor frequency and this firing occurs before the onset of the tremor which is recorded electromyographically. It is probable that the dopaminergic pathway from the substantia nigra to the corpus striatum exerts an inhibitory action since both levodopa and drugs which block central cholinergic muscarinic receptors have an effect in suppressing the symptoms of Parkinson's disease. It would seem likely that dopaminergic and cholinergic systems exist in opposition in the corpus striatum. In paralysis agitans and in post-encephalitic Parkinson's disease there is a reduction in dopaminergic function due to loss of transmitter. Reserpine may cause a Parkinsonian syndrome by depleting the cerebral tissues of catecholamines whereas the phenothiazine drugs may act by causing a competitive block of dopamine receptors.

Paralysis agitans is the commonest variety of Parkinson's disease with a prevalence probably in excess of one per 1000 of population (Schwab and England, 1958; Kurland, 1958; Brewis *et al.*, 1966). The aetiology remains unknown. Poskanzer and Schwab (1963), on the basis of its higher incidence in older age-groups, suggested that it might be due to exposure to an infective agent at the time of the worldwide outbreaks of encephalitis lethargica in the 1920s. However, Hoehn (1976) has shown that the age of onset has altered little since the end of the last century, and she concluded that paralysis agitans and post-encephalitic Parkinsonism were distinct entities. This is supported by the differing clinical features and natural history of the two disorders; thus in post-encephalitic Parkinson's disease the course is relatively non-progressive, associated symptoms such as tics and oculogyric crises may be a feature and the response to treatment with levodopa is frequently less favourable.

Where Parkinsonism is the result of a defined cause, such as medication with phenothiazines, treatment is primarily directed to removing the causative agent where this is possible. Sometimes, however, severely psychotic patients may require continued medication and in this event the symptoms may be relieved to some extent by administration of anticholinergic drugs. Levodopa, on the other hand, has relatively little effect on drug-induced Parkinsonism. In paralysis agitans treatment is directed to controlling the clinical features of tremor, rigidity and bradykinesia. At the present time medication with levodopa is the most effective measure available but unfortunately paralysis agitans is generally slowly progressive so that with the passage of time medication becomes less effective and the dosage needed to produce a therapeutic effect may be poorly tolerated. In a proportion of patients dementia also becomes a feature and this at present remains resistant to therapy (Pollock and Hornabrook, 1966).

LEVODOPA

The introduction of levodopa as an effective treatment for Parkinson's disease derives from the observation of Ehringer and Hornykiewicz in 1960 that the concentration of dopamine in the substantia nigra and corpus striatum of patients who had died of Parkinson's disease was markedly diminished in comparison with patients who had died from other causes. Dopamine, along with the other catecholamines, nor-adrenaline and 5-hydroxytryptamine, is probably a major chemical transmitter in the brain and there is a major dopaminergic pathway from the substantia nigra to the corpus striatum. Dopamine has been found to inhibit the majority of neurones in the caudate nucleus and is formed from the amino acid tyrosine which is converted to levodopa (L-3,4 dihydroxyphenylalanine) by tyrosine hydroxylase. The dopa is then converted to dopamine by the enzyme decarboxylase. The degra-dation of dopamine takes place by several pathways. In one it is con-verted by the enzyme dopamine β-hydroxylase to noradrenaline. A major part, however, is converted to homovanillic acid (HVA) and dihydroxyphenylacetic acid (DOPAC) both of which are excreted in the urine.

PHARMACOKINETICS

Levodopa is absorbed through the gastrointestinal tract, principally the jejunum, and is widely distributed throughout the body. Unlike dopa-mine it penetrates the blood—brain barrier. However, because much of it is decarboxylated to dopamine in the gut and the tissues, no more than 50 per cent reaches the circulation. Relatively large quantities must, therefore, be ingested to increase the concentrations in the central nervous system significantly. If levodopa is given together with a peripheral decarboxylase inhibitor such as L-α-methyldopa hydrazine (carbidopa) higher peak blood levels (1—3 μg/ml) are reached earlier and following lower oral doses. Lower doses are therefore more effec-tive in achieving significant concentrations in the nervous system. Levo-dopa itself has little pharmacological action but the catecholamines which are formed by its breakdown in the periphery may give rise to nausea, postural hypotension and cardiac arrhythmias and these side-effects are also diminished by the use of a peripheral decarboxylase inhibitor.

ADVERSE REACTIONS

The earliest side-effect of L-dopa is generally anorexia and nausea, and this effect may be lessened by taking the drug after meals. It is also lessened by giving the drug with a decarboxylase inhibitor so that the nausea may be partly the result of peripheral circulating dopamine al-though part of the effect may be centrally mediated. Other side-effects are postural hypotension, cardiac arrhythmias and psychiatric reactions which may range from a mild degree of euphoria or a disturbance of sleep pattern to confusional states and delirium. The most common adverse reaction limiting the dosage of levodopa which the patient will tolerate is dyskinesia, which may take the form of choreoathetoid involuntary movements. These effects are seldom seen when levodopa is given to healthy subjects. Initially they may consist of grimacing of the face or of mild peripheral movements such as curling of the toes but with increasing dosage may become widespread and severe. Other side-effects include hot flushes and pupillary dilatation and dark discoloration of urine, sweat or saliva. It has occasionally been known to precipitate gout. If given in association with monoamine oxidase inhibitors the combination may lead to possibly dangerous elevations of the blood pressure and the action of levodopa is blocked by pyridoxine which is a co-factor of dopa decarboxylase. If vitamin supplements are given to patients taking levodopa they should not therefore include pyridoxine, but this precaution is not necessary if levodopa is given along with a decarboxylase inhibitor (Klawans *et al.*, 1971). It is wise to withhold levodopa for a day or two before surgery as fluctuations in blood pressure may occur in association with anaesthesia.

TREATMENT WITH LEVODOPA

The initial observation of Birkmayer and Hornykiewicz (1961) that intravenous levodopa is effective in relieving the akinesia of Parkinson's disease has been amply confirmed by subsequent studies with oral preparations. Initially DL dopa was used but this carried a significant risk of side-effects, particularly marrow depression, and the levo isomer was found to be not only more effective but less toxic. Although the effect on tremor and rigidity is not always so marked as the effect on hypokinesia levodopa not infrequently benefits all the serious manifestations of Parkinson's disease and is at present the single most effective therapeutic agent in this condition.

If levodopa is given on its own it may be administered in an initial dose of 250 mg twice or three times a day which can be gradually and progressively increased to a level of 2—3 g daily, some patients benefiting from dosages as high as 4—5 g in the day. Because of the initial tendency to develop nausea, and the unpredictability of other side-effects such as psychiatric manifestations, it is generally wise to start with a very small dose increasing it gradually until a reasonable degree of benefit is achieved in the absence of side-effects. Involuntary movements are the most frequent and dose-limiting effects and there are some patients who will only tolerate comparatively low dosages without the development of involuntary movement. If movements develop these will generally diminish or cease if the dose is reduced.

The use of a decarboxylase inhibitor in association with levodopa makes it possible to treat the patient with substantially lower doses of levodopa and with markedly lower incidence of peripheral side-effects. Two decarboxylase inhibitors that are widely used are L-α-methyldopa hydrazine (carbidopa) and 1-DL seryl-2 (2,3,4 dihydroxybenzyl) hydrazine hydrochloride (benserazide) and these have become available in compound tablets, namely Sinemet which contains levodopa and carbidopa, and Madopar which contains levodopa and benserazide. Sinemet is made up in two strengths: Sinemet 275 containing 250 mg of levodopa and 25 mg of carbidopa, and Sinemet 110 containing 100 mg of levodopa and 10 mg of carbidopa. Madopar is made up as Madopar 250 containing 200 mg of levodopa and 50 mg of benserazide hydrochloride, and Madopar 125 containing 100 mg levodopa and 25 mg benserazide. The low-dose preparation Madopar 62.5 contains 50 mg levodopa and 12.5 mg benserazide. 100 mg of levodopa taken with a decarboxylase inhibitor is approximately equivalent to 500 mg of levodopa given on its own. In starting treatment with one of these preparations it is generally preferable to start with a low-dose preparation, gradually increasing the dose until optimum benefit is obtained. Although peripheral side-effects such as nausea and postural hypotension are less of a problem with these preparations, there is no difference in the incidence of central side-effects such as involuntary movements. Comparing preparations containing different decarboxylase inhibitors has shown little difference in overall effect but some patients find one preparation preferable.

When treatment with levodopa is initiated it may be a week or a fortnight before significant benefit is obtained. Although it produces marked symptomatic benefit it does not appear to arrest the progress of the disorder. In some patients the benefit is comparatively short-lived but many achieve significant improvement over 5 years or longer, although as time goes on they may require increasing dosage to achieve the same benefit. On the other hand, the ability to tolerate adequate dosage may be restricted by the development of side-effects and a reduction in dosage may sometimes be beneficial. Thus involuntary movements may not be present as a side-effect when treatment is started but may become an increasing problem with long-term therapy. A particularly troublesome late effect is that improvement may give way to oscillation in performance leading eventually to the so-called 'on/off' phenomenon. In some patients the 'on/off' effect occurs as a sudden accentuation of bradykinesia so that the patient becomes totally unable to move; this condition lasts from a few minutes to several hours, and again ceases relatively suddenly. In others the situation is complicated by involuntary movements which occur intermittently and may become so pronounced as to make gait almost impossible. In some patients the 'on/off' effect may be relieved by giving levodopa in small doses at frequent intervals. In others cessation of levodopa therapy for several weeks, possibly accompanied by the substitution of amantadine or anticholinergic drugs, may make it possible for treatment with levodopa to be restarted with increased benefit and diminished side-effects (Yahr and Duvoisin, 1972).

Levodopa is of most benefit in paralysis agitans and although it may be helpful in post-encephalitic Parkinson's disease it is less effective and less well tolerated. In Parkinson's disease associated with syndromes such as progressive supranuclear palsy (Steele—Richardson syndrome) or olivo-ponto cerebellar degeneration the effect may be disappointing and it does not benefit drug-induced Parkinsonism following medication with reserpine or the phenothiazines. In the very elderly, or in patients with dementia or a history of psychiatric disturbance, very great caution must be exercised in initiating therapy with levodopa.

How far it is advisable to initiate therapy with levodopa in the mild early case remains uncertain. On the one hand there may be an advantage in initiating effective treatment early; alternatively it has been held that to start with anticholinergic drugs alone or with amantadine may delay the development of long-term side-effects of levodopa. There may therefore be a case for withholding levodopa until there is significant impairment of function.

ANTICHOLINERGIC DRUGS

Anticholinergic drugs were introduced more than 100 years ago and Ordenstein (1867) in his MD thesis refers to the early use by Charcot of hyoscyamine in Parkinson's disease. Stramonium, atropine and hyoscine were widely used until 1947 when a variety of synthetic anticholinergic drugs were introduced (*see* Table 4.1). These drugs block muscarinic receptors for acetylcholine in the central nervous system and it is probable that their therapeutic action is due to blocking of cholinergic effects in the striatum which oppose the action of dopamine. However, there is some evidence also that anticholinergic drugs inhibit the re-uptake of dopamine in dopaminergic nerve fibres. These drugs produce some benefit in tremor and rigidity but are less effective in controlling bradykinesia. Some of the synthetic anticholinergic drugs also have antihistaminic actions but it is doubtful if these are significant

Table 4.1   Anticholinergic drugs used in Parkinson's disease

Drug	Preparation	Dosage
Benapryzine	Brizin 50 mg tabs.	50 mg 3 or 4 times daily
Benzhexol	Artane 2 mg and 5 mg scored tabs.	1 mg first day increasing gradually to 5—15 mg per day
Benztropine mesylate	Cogentin 2 mg quarter scored tabs.	0.5 mg per day increasing by 0.5 mg every 6 days to maximum of 6 mg per day
Biperiden hydrochloride	Akineton 2 mg scored tabs.	1 mg twice daily initially increasing gradually to 2 mg three times daily
Chlorphenoxamine hydrochloride	Clorevan 50 mg tabs.	50—100 mg three times daily
Methixene hydrochloride	Tremonil 5 mg scored tabs.	2.5 mg three times daily increasing to 5—10 mg three times daily
Orphenadrine hydrochloride	Disipal 50 mg tabs.	50 mg three times daily increasing to 100 mg three times daily
Procyclidine hydrochloride	Kemadrin 5 mg scored tabs.	2.5 mg three times daily increasing to 5—10 mg three times daily

in relation to their anti-Parkinsonian effects. Unlike levodopa anticholinergic drugs are also effective in drug-induced Parkinsonism. Some, such as orphenadrine, have a mild euphoriant action which may also be helpful. They may be given with benefit in association with levodopa, the combination of drugs sometimes being more effective than either drug taken singly (Hughes *et al.*, 1971), but caution has to be exercised in patients who develop involuntary movements as side-effects of levodopa as these involuntary movements may sometimes be aggravated by anticholinergic drugs. Side-effects of anticholinergic drugs include failure of ocular accommodation, pupillary dilatation, dry mouth, constipation and urinary retention, and patients, particularly the elderly, with arteriosclerosis may suffer confusional episodes and hallucinations during the night. If anticholinergic drugs are discontinued it is important to do this gradually as sometimes a very marked exacerbation of bradykinesia and rigidity occurs following sudden withdrawal.

AMANTADINE

Amantadine is an antiviral agent which is effective against influenza and its value in Parkinson's disease was discovered by chance when it was used as an antiviral agent on a patient with Parkinson's disease (Schwab and England, 1969). Although its mode of action is not understood its effects are similar to those of levodopa although less pronounced, and it is possible that it may act either by increasing the release or inhibiting the re-uptake of dopamine. It is made up in tablets of 100 mg which may be given twice daily starting with a single tablet on the first day. Adverse reactions include psychiatric disturbances, but these are uncommon and milder side-effects such as livedo reticularis and peripheral oedema are not necessarily indications for discontinuing the drug. Unfortunately, though patients who are moderately affected by Parkinson's disease may develop considerable and useful benefit, the benefit is not always well sustained and the effects may appear to wear off after a period of weeks or months. It may be given along with anticholinergic drugs or with levodopa but it is perhaps particularly valuable as an alternative to levodopa and can be given during periods when that drug is discontinued.

BROMOCRIPTINE

The failure of levodopa to halt the progression of Parkinson's disease and the development of drug-induced side-effects with prolonged therapy such as involuntary movements, the 'on/off' effect and psychiatric disturbances seriously limit its value as a single mode of treatment. Drugs which stimulate dopamine receptors in the corpus striatum might also be expected to relieve the symptoms of Parkinson's disease and this has been found to be the case with apomorphine. This drug, however, has such a short duration of action, and its side-effects are so distressing, that it has not found any place in therapy. Other dopaminergic agonists include piribdil, ergotrile and bromocriptine but the use of the first two of these preparations is also restricted by side-effects. Bromocriptine, however, which is an ergolene derivative, stimulates postsynaptic dopamine receptors and has been found to be effective in relieving the symptoms of Parkinson's disease. Unfortunately, it also gives rise to side-effects similar to those of levodopa, namely involuntary movements and in some patients very distressing psychiatric disturbances may occur. It is available in 2.5 and 10 mg tablets and it is advisable to start with 2.5 mg in the day which may be increased by 2.5 mg twice a week up to 40 mg in the day if the patient will tolerate this amount. It is best taken after meals and may be effectively administered in divided doses three or four times in the day. If given initially to untreated patients its effects appear to be similar to those of levodopa but it is doubtful if in this situation it has any advantage over levodopa and it is considerably more expensive. In patients who have been treated with levodopa, and where the effect of levodopa is appearing to diminish or where there are severe side-effects or an 'on/off' effect, partial replacement of levodopa with a low dose of bromocriptine may sometimes improve control although its effect on the 'on/off' effect is disappointing. 5–10 mg of bromocriptine is approximately equivalent to 500 mg of levodopa without a decarboxylase inhibitor. Patients who are unable to tolerate levodopa or who do not respond to it seldom benefit from bromocriptine (Parkes *et al.*, 1976; Godwin-Austin and Smith, 1977).

AMPHETAMINES AND OTHER DRUGS

Amphetamine has a limited action in the relief of Parkinsonian symptoms and in the past has been widely used particularly in postencephalitic Parkinson's disease where it may reduce the frequency of oculogyric crises. Its action is by blocking the re-uptake and promoting the release of catecholamines from presynaptic terminals of central neurones and Parkes *et al.* (1975) consider that its relatively limited clinical effect may be due to the already depleted state of central neurones in Parkinson's disease.

Tricyclic antidepressants such as imiprimine or desiprimine have also been used. These are useful in alleviating co-existing depression in addition to a mild anti-Parkinsonian effect. Their main action is by preventing the re-uptake of noradrenaline but their anticholinergic effect may also be helpful.

In a number of patients with Parkinson's disease action tremor in addition to tremor at rest is a feature (Lance *et al.*, 1963). In these patients it may be helpful to give a β-blocking agent such as propranolol in a dose of 60–120 mg per day (*see* Chapter 5).

Monoamine oxidase inhibitors have a weak anti-Parkinsonian effect and may potentiate the action of levodopa but their use is not recommended on account of the risk of producing a hypertensive reaction (Hunter *et al.*, 1970). Deprenil (phenylisopropylmethylpropinylamine HCl) specifically blocks the action of monoamine oxidase B which deaminates phenylethylamine and benzylamine in contradistinction to monoamine oxidase A which inactivates noradrenaline and 5-hydroxytryptamine, and early trials suggest that its use in conjunction with levodopa and a decarboxylase inhibitor may be helpful particularly in patients subject to an 'on/off' effect (Birkmayer *et al.*, 1977; Lees *et al.*, 1977).

SURGICAL TREATMENT

Although early studies involving destruction of part of the internal capsule have been found to be effective in the relief of rigidity and tremor in Parkinson's disease effective surgical treatment dates from the discovery that lesions in the globus pallidus and ansa lenticularis, and subsequently the lateral ventral nucleus of the thalamus, were effective in relieving tremor and rigidity. This knowledge followed Cooper's (1954) serendipitous discovery that improvement in tremor and rigidity followed ligation of the anterior choroidal artery. Unfortunately, although surgical lesions produced a marked decrease in tremor and rigidity, they had little effect on bradykinesia which was sometimes aggravated after surgery; it likewise had no effect on the natural progression of the disease. Since the introduction of levodopa fewer operations for Parkinson's disease have been carried out and it would appear now that surgical treatment is seldom indicated except possibly in the case of a patient with severe tremor unresponsive to medical treatment and with little accompanying bradykinesia.

GENERAL MEASURES

Although specific drug therapy may do much to relieve the disability in many patients with Parkinson's disease, relief from therapy is often incomplete and general supportive measures are frequently indicated. Alterations to a person's house to make it suitable for a patient with disability are frequently necessary and include suitably placed rails beside steps and in the toilet; this is particularly necessary if the patients have difficulty with postural control, as is often the case when the disease is advanced. If patients find it difficult to turn in bed a firmer mattress may help. Holding a cup may be difficult because of tremor, and straws may be used to overcome this difficulty; special cutlery may be provided by the local Health and Social Services departments. Physiotherapy in hospital may be helpful in improving a patient's posture and gait. Constipation may be a problem and may be helped by adequate roughage in the diet, by regular exercise and, if necessary, by bulk laxatives. Parkinson's disease is a condition which may affect a patient's ability to drive a car, and the development of Parkinson's disease is one condition where the holder of a driving licence in the United Kingdom is required to report the condition to the licensing centre; renewal of a driving licence may depend on the submission of appropriate medical information.

An appreciable number of patients with Parkinson's disease develop dementia. In this situation medication is less effective and side-effects more readily develop. General measures become very important and are discussed further in Chapter 8.

REFERENCES

Birkmayer, W and Hornykiewicz, O (1961) Der L-3,4-Dioxyphenylalanine (= DOPA) — Effekt bei der Parkinson-Akinese. *Wiener Klinische Wochenschrift,* **73**, 787—788.

Birkmayer, W, Riederer, P, Ambrozi, L and Youdim, M B H (1977) Implications of combined treatment with madopar and L-deprenil in Parkinson's disease, a long-term study. *Lancet,* **1**, 439—443.

Brewis, M, Poskanzer, D C, Rolland, C and Miller, H (1966) Neurological disease in an English city. *Acta Neurologica Scandinavica,* **42**, *Suppl.* 24, 1—89.

Cooper, I S (1954) Surgical occlusion of anterior choroidal artery in Parkinsonism. *Surgery, Gynaecology and Obstetrics,* **99**, 207—219.

Ehringer, H and Hornykiewicz, O (1960) Distribution of noradrenaline and dopamine (3-hydroxytyramine) in the human brain and their behaviour in disease of the extrapyramidal system. *Wiener Klinische Wochenschrift,* **38**, 1236—1239.

Godwin-Austin, R D and Smith, N S (1977) Comparison of the effects of bromocriptine and levodopa in Parkinson's disease. *Journal of Neurology, Neurosurgery and Psychiatry,* **40**, 479—482.

Hoehn, M M (1976) Age distribution of patients with Parkinsonism. *Journal of the American Geriatric Society,* **24**, 79—85.

Hughes, R C, Polgar, J G, Weightman, D and Walton, J N (1971) Levodopa in Parkinsonism: the effects of withdrawal of anticholinergic drugs. *British Medical Journal,* **2**, 487.

Hunter, K R, Boakes, A J, Laurence, D R and Stern, G M (1970) Monoamine oxidase inhibitors and L-dopa. *British Medical Journal,* **3**, 388.

Klawans, H L Jr, Ringel, S P and Shenker, D (1971) Failure of vitamin B6 to reduce the L-dopa effect in patients on a dopa decarboxylase inhibitor. *Journal of Neurology, Neurosurgery and Psychiatry,* **34**, 682—686.

Kurland, I J (1958) Descriptive epidemiology of selected neurologic and myopathic disorders with particular relevance to a survey in Rochester, Minnesota. *Journal of Chronic Diseases,* **8**, 378—418.

Lance, J W, Schwab, R S and Peterson, E A (1963) Action tremor and the cogwheel phenomenon in Parkinson's disease. *Brain,* **86**, 95—110.

Lees, A J, Kohout, L J and Shaw, K W (1977) Deprenil in Parkinson's disease. *Lancet*, **2**, 791.

Ordenstein, L (1867) Sur la Parelysie Agitante et la sclérose en plaques géneralisée. Thèse pour le doctorat en medecine. Paris: Martinet.

Parkes, J D, Marsden, C D, Donaldson, I, Galea-Debono, A, Walters, J, Kennedy, G and Asselman, P (1976) Bromocriptine treatment in Parkinson's disease. *Journal of Neurology, Neurosurgery and Psychiatry*, **39**, 232–237.

Parkes, J D, Tarsy, D, Marsden, C D, Bovill, K T, Phipps, J A, Rose, P and Asselmen, P (1975) Amphetamines and the treatment of Parkinson's disease. *Journal of Neurology, Neurosurgery and Psychiatry*, **38**, 232–237.

Pollock, M and Hornabrook, R W (1966) The prevalence, natural history and dementia of Parkinson's disease. *Brain*, **89**, 429–448.

Poskanzer, D C and Schwab, R S (1963) Cohort analysis of Parkinson's syndrome: evidence for a single aetiology related to subclinical infection about 1920. *Journal of Chronic Diseases*, **16**, 961–973.

Schwab, R S and England, A C (1958) Parkinson's disease. *Journal of Chronic Diseases*, **8**, 488–509.

Schwab, R S and England, A C (1969) Amantadine HCl (symmetrical) and its relation to Levo-Dopa in the treatment of Parkinson's disease. *Transactions of the American Neurological Association*, **94**, 85–90.

Yahr, M D and Duvoisin, R C (1972) Drug therapy of Parkinsonism. *New England Journal of Medicine*, **287**, 20–24.

CHAPTER FIVE

Involuntary Movement Disorders

It is of interest that a major side-effect of levodopa when given to patients with Parkinson's disease is the production of involuntary movements similar in character to those seen in movement disorders such as chorea. This would appear to suggest that other movement disorders in addition to Parkinson's disease may be related to an imbalance between the activity of different chemical transmitters mediating the output of different systems concerned in the control of movement. Apart from this general concept, however, little is known regarding the pharmacology underlying movement disorders, although it is known that in Huntington's chorea the brain is depleted of γ-aminobutyric acid (GABA) and the enzyme concerned with its formation, glutamic acid decarboxylase (Perry *et al.*, 1973; Bird *et al.*, 1973). It is also known that in hepatolenticular degeneration (Wilson's disease), the treatment of which is discussed in a later section, a disorder of movement is the result of injury to the basal ganglia by deposition of copper within its structure. In general it has been found that drugs which deplete the brain of catecholamines, such as reserpine or tetrabenazine, and drugs which block the action of dopamine at its receptor site, such as phenothiazines, butyrophenones and pimozide, are effective in relieving choreoathetosis and to a lesser degree dystonia. Phenothiazines, however, can also produce acute dystonic reactions which settle if the drug is withdrawn and also involuntary movements affecting particularly the face and mouth, which may persist after withdrawal of the drug. The mechanism of these effects is not known although it has been suggested that continuous use of phenothiazines may lead to denervation hypersensitivity at dopaminergic synapses (Klawans, 1973). In certain disorders of movement such as tics, hemifacial spasm, torticollis and writer's cramp no definite organic pathology has been described and it is uncertain to what extent these disorders are organically determined and how far they are influenced by psychological factors. Myoclonus is sometimes difficult to distinguish from other varieties of movement disorder. It is essentially a sudden movement which is involuntary and may occur in healthy subjects as a jerking of the limbs particularly on falling asleep. It may represent a local discharge of nerve cells either from the brain or spinal cord, in which case it may be the result of anoxic damage. It is also a frequent manifestation of epilepsy.

DRUG THERAPIES

Tetrabenazine

This drug is similar in its action to reserpine which depletes the brain of catecholamines and 5-hydroxytryptamine, but its action is more rapid and of shorter duration. It is made up in 25 mg tablets (Nitoman) and may be given in an initial dose of 25 mg once or twice a day, gradually increasing by 25 mg increments every three or four days. Up to 200 mg a day may be given but a satisfactory maintenance dose is generally of the order of 75—100 mg per day. It is effective principally in the treatment of choreiform movements. Side-effects include mild digestive upset, hypotension, drowsiness and Parkinsonian features, but the most serious limiting effect is depression which can gradually develop if treatment is continued for an extended period of time.

Haloperidol

This drug is a butyrophenone and like the phenothiazines is effective in the control of psychotic states. It may be used in the treatment of choreiform movements and is effective in the control of motor tics including the syndrome of Gilles de la Tourette. It is rapidly absorbed, reaching a peak level in about 4 h with a half-life of less than 24 h. It may be given with an initial dose of 0.5 mg three times a day gradually increasing until an adequate effect is achieved, generally with a dose of 4—6 mg per day although in some patients doses of 10 mg or greater may be required. Side-effects include drowsiness and hypotension and the drug may increase the intra-ocular pressure. It can also give rise to Parkinsonism, akathisia and to acute dystonic reactions.

Pimozide

This drug is a diphenylbutyl piperidine. It has powerful antipsychotic properties and is also effective in the control of choreiform movements.

It is readily absorbed but only a small proportion penetrates the blood—brain barrier. It is made up in 2 mg tablets and may be given in an initial dose of one tablet daily increasing gradually up to a maximum of about 10 mg per day. Side-effects include drowsiness, and Parkinsonism may occur with high dosage.

Phenothiazines

This group of drugs, major tranquillisers effective in the control of psychotic states, are also effective in the control of choreiform movements. Chlorpromazine is made up in 25 mg tablets and may be given in an initial dose of 25 mg three times a day increasing if necessary to 100—200 mg per day. It is rapidly absorbed and distributed throughout the body. Side-effects include sedation, hypotension, seizures, photosensitivity and Parkinsonism. Jaundice is an occasional hypersensitivity reaction. Thiopropazate is a phenothiazine which has been widely used for the control of choreiform movements; it is made up in 5 mg tablets and may be given in a dosage of 15—20 mg per day.

Benzodiazapines

This group contains a number of drugs which have sedative, tranquillising, anticonvulsant and muscle-relaxant properties. Diazepam is absorbed readily by mouth, rapidly crossing the blood—brain barrier. There is a wide variation between the plasma levels obtained in different individuals with the same dosage. Initial dosage may be 2 mg three times a day increasing gradually, but when levels of 5—10 mg per day are reached drowsiness may be a limiting factor. It has a limited place in the management of involuntary movements but may be of benefit in the treatment of torticollis and torsion dystonia. Clonazepam is similar in many respects to diazepam but is particularly liable to cause drowsiness unless the dosage is very gradually built up. It is made up in 0.5 mg tablets and 2 mg tablets, and an initial dose might be 0.5 mg per day increasing gradually to between 4 and 8 mg per day. Its main therapeutic indication is in the treatment of epilepsy and in the treatment of dyskinesias its main value is in the control of myoclonus.

CLINICAL PROBLEMS AND THE RESULTS OF TREATMENT

1. Chorea

Choreiform movements occur in a variety of disorders including in particular Sydenham's and Huntington's chorea; they may also be seen less commonly in association with conditions such as thyrotoxicosis and systemic lupus erythematosus. The general management of Huntington's chorea is discussed in Chapter 11. Drugs which are effective in the control of choreiform movements include tetrabenazine, haloperidol, pimozide and phenothiazines. Where chorea occurs in association with thyrotoxicosis it will generally resolve with treatment of the thyroid disorder. In Sydenham's chorea it is generally relatively easily controlled with haloperidol or with a phenothiazine drug. In a progressive condition such as Huntington's chorea control may be very difficult, and drugs such as haloperidol or chlorpromazine may only be effective in dosage high enough to give rise to side-effects. In this situation tetrabenazine may be of value but again the hazard of depression is a serious limiting factor if treatment is prolonged.

2. Hemiballismus

Hemiballismus or hemichorea may occur as a result of a lesion, generally vascular, affecting the contralateral subthalamic nucleus. It may occur as an isolated event or in association with an acute hemiplegia, and is an occasional complication of stereotactic thalamotomy. The movements may be extremely violent and exhausting so that although the natural tendency is for recovery slowly to take place the condition may be fatal unless treatment is instituted. Tetrabenazine, haloperidol or the phenothiazines may all be effective but if the condition does not respond to medication contralateral thalamotomy may be considered.

3. Dystonia and athetosis

Dystonia is a fixed attitude of the body in which there is sustained contraction of the muscles maintaining the abnormal posture; in athetosis the limbs or body move from one dystonic posture to another. A dystonic posture is frequently seen in advanced Parkinson's disease and athetosis occurs most commonly as part of athetoid cerebral palsy. Torsion dystonia is seen in its most severe form in the hereditary condition of dystonia musculorum deformans. Choreiform movements become slow and increase in amplitude, and they may take on the character of athetosis so that one may speak of choreoathetosis. Torsion dystonia and athetoid cerebral palsy may each be associated with pathology affecting the basal ganglia; in particular, cavitation in the putamen. Acute dystonia may also occur in patients receiving treatment with phenothiazines or haloperidol. This generally occurs in children or in young adults and the abnormalities of movement may include oculogyric crisis, retrocollis or opisthotonos.

Treatment of torsion dystonia is difficult and unsatisfactory. Some limited response may be obtained with phenothiazines, haloperidol or tetrabenazine but other patients may benefit more from large doses of diazepam or anticholinergic drugs such as benzhexol hydrochloride. Stereotactic surgery (Cooper, 1970) has been attempted in a number of patients but the results are frequently unrewarding. Acute dystonia precipitated by phenothiazines generally ceases when the drug is withdrawn and in the acute state may be treated effectively by diazepam (10 mg i.v.) or by an anticholinergic drug (benztropine 2 mg i.v.).

4. Torticollis

In this condition muscle spasm leads to twisting of the neck to either side or backwards (retrocollis). The condition tends to be slowly progressive over the years but in some the condition appears to arrest and in a few cases spontaneous remission appears to occur. No pathological lesion has been found in the brain. Some cases have appeared to follow psychological stress (Paterson, 1945) but consistent psychological factors have not been identified (Herz and Glaser, 1949; Cockburn, 1971). Treatment with drugs is on the whole unsatisfactory although some improvement has been obtained with diazepam, phenothiazines, haloperidol or amantadine. Psychotherapy (Paterson, 1945) has had its advocates but in general has had little success. Stereotactic surgery (Cooper, 1964) has been carried out on a number of patients but the most effective surgical treatment has involved selective unilateral section of the accessory nerve and of the upper cervical roots. This procedure, however, may likewise only give partial relief.

5. Orofacial dyskinesia

Grimacing movements of the mouth and tongue may occur as one of the varieties of involuntary movement seen in patients with Parkinson's disease as a side-effect of therapy with levodopa. It is also seen occasionally in elderly people but it occurs as a serious complication of long-term therapy with phenothiazines particularly when these drugs are given in high dosage to elderly patients with psychiatric disorders. In this situation the condition is referred to as *tardive dyskinesia*. It continues after cessation of the medication and may be relieved by tetrabenazine or by increasing the dose of the phenothiazine drug. Possible underlying mechanisms include denervation hypersensitivity of dopamine receptors, excessive synthesis or reduced presynaptic re-uptake of dopamine or an imbalance between cholinergic or dopaminergic transmitter systems (Klawans, 1973). Treatment is made difficult by the need which may be present to continue medication for the psychiatric condition for which the patient is having treatment, but it is desirable to discontinue the drug which has precipitated the symptom if this is possible. Pimozide, which has a selective blocking action on dopamine receptors, may have a place in treatment (Claveria *et al.*, 1975). Prevention should be directed to limiting where possible the long-term use of phenothiazines in high dosage for elderly patients. Concurrent use of anticholinergic drugs appears to increase the risk of tardive dyskinesia developing.

6. Essential tremor

This tremor, unlike that of Parkinson's disease, appears in the hands on maintaining a posture and is not present at rest. It does not disappear with movement and it often interferes with simple tasks such as holding a cup and saucer or writing, and electromyographic studies show that the recruitment order of motor units is disturbed and there may be simultaneous contraction of agonist and antagonist muscles. There is a strong familial tendency and in some families the condition is inherited as an autosomal dominant trait. Sometimes it is associated with titubation of the head and tremor of the jaw. A number of patients notice that a drink containing alcohol will bring about temporary relief but drug therapy is not altogether satisfactory. Some patients obtain relief from regular medication with diazepam. The most effective single remedy appears to be the β-adrenergic blocking agent propranolol. This may be taken in a dose of 60—120 mg daily; however, some patients find it more satisfactory not to take regular medication but to reserve the drug for occasions when the tremor is likely to prove a particular embarrassment.

7. Tics and myoclonus

A tic is a stereotyped movement which occurs from time to time with the same characteristics at the same site. It may involve a facial movement such as eye-blinking or grimacing, and sometimes the limbs or trunk are involved. It occurs particularly in children and particularly if they are emotionally disturbed; frequently, but not always, the tics tend to settle down as the child reaches adult life. They may be associated sometimes with other obsessional characteristics and with compulsive utterances. Generally treatment is not necessary and all that may be required is supportive psychotherapy. The syndrome of Gilles de la Tourette is one which occurs in childhood or adolescence in which stereotyped movements take place periodically and which, as the condition progresses, become associated with abnormal noises such as coughs or barks and later the muttering of obscene utterances. Many of these patients recover as they grow up, and treatment with haloperidol may bring partial or complete relief.

In myoclonus the repetitive muscle jerks lack the stereotyped character of the compulsive tic. Myoclonic jerks occur frequently in association with epilepsy and the treatment of myoclonus in this setting has been discussed in Chapter 2. Essential myoclonus is a condition which is sometimes familial, with an autosomal dominant inheritance in which periodic myoclonic jerks of the trunk and limbs occur without any sign of epilepsy or of neurological disease. Myoclonus, when it is a disabling symptom, may be relieved by benzodiazepines such as clonazepam and also sometimes by sodium valproate.

8. Hemifacial spasm

In this condition the patient develops irregular twitching of the muscles, initially around one eye, subsequently spreading to involve the whole of one side of the face. It is restricted to the territory of the facial nerve and generally no underlying cause can be discovered although sometimes it may follow Bell's palsy. Treatment with drugs is unsatisfactory although diazepam may give some symptomatic relief; selective division of the terminal endings of the facial nerve may give relief although at the expense of causing a degree of facial weakness.

9. Writer's cramp

This condition has been characterised as an occupational palsy and the term can only be strictly applied when the disability affects a single action only without other evidence of inco-ordination or neurological disorder. Not uncommonly writer's cramp can be the first sign of spastic weakness in the hand, Parkinson's disease or torsion dystonia; but if this is the case other actions in addition to writing may come to be affected. In general the prognosis is unfavourable and psychological treatment is frequently ineffective. Liversedge and Sylvester (1955) obtained improvement in a group of patients by the use of a deconditioning procedure in which a special apparatus was used which allowed electric shocks to be delivered to the left hand whenever the pen strayed from its course. Experience with this treatment, however, is very limited.

REFERENCES

Bird, E D, MacKay, A V P, Rayner, C N and Iversen, L L (1973) Reduced glutamic-acid-decarboxylase activity of post-mortem brain in Huntington's chorea. *Lancet*, 1, 1090—1092.

Claveria, L E, Teychenne, P F, Calne, D B, Haskayne, L, Petrie, A, Pallis, C A and Lodge-Patch, I C (1975) Tardive dyskinesia treated with pimozide. *Journal of the Neurological Sciences*, 24, 393—401.

Cockburn, J J (1971) Spasmodic torticollis: a psychogenic condition? *Journal of Psychosomatic Research*, 15, 471—477.

Cooper, I S (1964) Effect of thalamic lesions upon torticollis. *New England Journal of Medicine*, 270, 967—972.

Cooper, I S (1970) Neurosurgical treatment of dystonia. *Neurology*, 20, (2), 133—148.

Herz, F and Glaser, G H (1949) Spasmodic torticollis. II. Clinical evaluation. *Archives of Neurology and Psychiatry*, 61, 227—239.

Klawans, H (1973) The pharmacology of tardive dyskinesias. *American Journal of Psychiatry*, 130, 82—86.

Liversedge, L A and Sylvester, J D (1955) Conditioning techniques in the treatment of writer's cramp. *Lancet*, 1, 1147—1149.

Paterson, M T (1945) Spasmodic torticollis: results of psychotherapy in twenty-one cases. *Lancet*, 2, 556—559.

Perry, T L, Hansen, S and Kloster, M (1973) Huntington's chorea: deficiency of gamma-aminobutyric acid in the brain. *New England Journal of Medicine*, 288, 337—342.

CHAPTER SIX

Chronic or Recurrent Pain

BASIC MECHANISMS IN RELATION TO TREATMENT

Recent biochemical and physiological research is just beginning to unravel the complex mechanisms in the central control of pain. The input to the spinal cord of information concerning noxious stimuli is largely conducted in unmyelinated C-fibres with some input from small myelinated fibres. These small fibres, together with large sensory afferent fibres, terminate in the dorsal horn of the grey matter of the spinal cord in complex laminae (Rexed's laminae). The interaction between large and small fibres projecting to the cord appears to be important in controlling pain. The large fibre inputs from cutaneous endings have an inhibitory effect on the perception of pain. Enhancement of this inhibitory effect may be the basis for traditional pain-relieving manoeuvres such as rubbing an adjacent part, as these increase the non-painful cutaneous input. Transcutaneous nerve stimulation, and perhaps acupuncture, may act by similar mechanisms. The axons in the posterior columns have segmental collaterals which also inhibit pain-perception, and it is likely that increase in activity in these fibres occurs during dorsal column stimulation for pain relief. The spinothalamic pathways arise in the dorsal horns and conduct information giving clear localisation of the site of pain. This pathway relays in the thalamus and projects mainly to the parietal cortex. It is divided in cordotomy for the relief of pain. Other projections from the dorsal horn form the spinoreticular pathways. These have complex connections in the reticular formation, and thereafter diffusely to the thalamus, hypothalamus and the cortex. Stimulation of these pathways in the ventrolateral periaqueductal cells may relieve pain promptly by activation of descending pathways to the dorsal horn. These descending inhibitory pathways include 5-hydroxytryptamine-containing cells from the raphe nucleus and noradrenaline-containing cells of the locus coeruleus. It is possible that the alleviation of pain in some patients treated with tricyclic antidepressants is by inhibition of the re-uptake of monoamines released from the terminations of these pathways. In addition, opiate receptors in the dorsal horn and periaqueductal cells may be involved in the control of pain. The role of other putative neurotransmitter systems is uncertain. Psychological factors contribute greatly to the perception of pain which is increased by anxiety, depression and lack of support from those caring for the patient. In addition, pain is influenced by the situation in which it occurs; often it is greater in civilian injuries than in war, more in chronic ill-health than after an operation producing acute pain, and sometimes more when litigation is pending.

TREATMENT

1. General management

Chronic pain is demoralising. Its relief must involve consideration of both the nature of the pain, and the patient. The cause of the pain should be clearly identified in each patient. Thus, for example, a patient with known malignant disease may have pain arising from other causes which require separate treatment and the pain should not be assumed to be a direct consequence of the tumour. Anxiety and fear, depression, anger, inadequate sleep and nutrition may exacerbate chronic pain. Accompanying symptoms such as nausea, vomiting or cough should be treated. The pain may fluctuate during the day.

Pain often arises from abnormal stimuli perceived by a normal nervous system, e.g. inflammatory joint disease, cardiac pain, smooth muscle spasm, and malignant disease. Obviously the underlying disease should be treated if possible. Sometimes local heat, massage or rest is helpful. With severe, persistent pain, as with malignant disease or where the pain arises from disorders in the nervous system, the aim of treatment is to modify the response of the nervous system to the pain either by drugs, selective lesions, or stimulation. The care of patients in chronic pain has improved in recent years with two organisational developments. Pain clinics are now held in many hospitals, staffed by anaesthetists, neurologists, neurosurgeons, or others committed to the relief of pain. Special expertise develops in these clinics and they are to be encouraged. The other development is the provision of specialised units for the care of patients with terminal malignant disease where management at home is inappropriate. These are often hospices or wards which provide humane care in which compassion is combined with skill in using drugs and other pain-relieving techniques.

2. Psychological factors in pain

The physician dealing with chronic pain should attempt to distinguish three situations which are important in the management of the patient.

(1) Pain of psychiatric origin, most commonly depression or anxiety. The primary treatment here is of the underlying depression, anxiety or neuroticism usually by simple psychotherapy. Antidepressants, benzodiazepines, and phenothiazines are used as required. Some patients may have hysterical personality traits or hysterical conversion syndromes.

(2) Psychological factors exacerbating organic pain. When a psychiatric disorder, e.g. depression or an anxiety state, exacerbates organic pain both the organic and the psychological factors have to be recognised and treated. This group may be difficult to separate from the third category.

(3) Psychological effects of chronic pain. Chronic pain often produces a variety of psychological disturbances with the development of depression, apathy, anxiety, irritability, and aggression. The primary aim is to relieve the organic pain but understanding of the patient with psychological symptoms is required.

3. Drug treatment

The choice of analgesic drugs is determined by whether a mild, moderate or potent analgesic is required, whether anti-inflammatory, antipyretic, sedative or euphoriant effects are needed, and the preferred route of administration. Parenteral medication should be avoided for chronic pain where possible.

It is very important that medication should be given sufficiently regularly to prevent the re-emergence of pain. Drugs should not be given 'as required', i.e. withheld until the pain has reached unacceptable levels, probably several times each day; instead, the drugs should be given on a regular basis to prevent the re-emergence of chronic pain. In addition to analgesics, the use of hypnotics, tranquillisers, antidepressants and anticonvulsants may be considered.

(a) Mild analgesics

Most patients have already tried mild analgesics. These all exhibit a ceiling effect for analgesia, i.e. analgesia which is not increased with further doses of the drug although adverse effects may increase. Paracetamol is a mild analgesic and antipyretic without anti-inflammatory effects. It has a short half-life of about 2 h, and should be administered in 500–1000 mg doses up to six times daily. Gastric bleeding and dyspepsia are not problems.

Aspirin has anti-inflammatory effects as well as analgesic and anti-pyretic actions. It is particularly valuable in metastatic bone pain where prostaglandins may contribute to pain. It is not useful, however, for visceral pain arising from gastrointestinal, or genitourinary systems, or from the heart. The dose is 300–900 mg, given up to 4-hourly. Gastric erosions may occur at low dose, and are only partially avoided with enteric-coated preparations. Tinnitus and dizziness occur at higher doses.

Indomethacin is a useful analgesic drug with anti-inflammatory properties and, like aspirin, may produce gastric ulceration. The initial dose is 25 mg b.d., gradually increasing the dose to achieve pain relief.

Mefenamic acid (Ponstan) and flufenamic acid (Meralen) also have analgesic and anti-inflammatory effects. They are given in doses of 250–500 mg orally q.i.d. and 200 mg q.i.d. respectively.

Codeine (methylmorphine) has mild analgesic effects, and may also be used to control cough and diarrhoea. It may be given as codeine phosphate in doses ranging from 10 to 60 mg 4-hourly. Constipation is the major side-effect. Dihydrocodeine (DF118) is a derivative of codeine with more potent effects and similar adverse effects. Habituation occurs with regular treatment. It is given in 30–60 mg doses.

Dextropropoxyphene is a mild narcotic analgesic, structurally related to methadone, but it does not have useful actions in suppressing cough. In the UK it is marketed as dextropropoxyphene hydrochloride 32.5 mg with paracetamol 325 mg as 'distalgesic'. Other mild narcotic analgesics, without proven superiority, are pholcodeine, dextromethorphan, hydromorphone, dipipanone, anileridine, ethoheptazine, and methyl-dihydromorphinone.

(b) Narcotic analgesics

Morphia and heroin are potent analgesic drugs with additional sedative, anxiolytic or euphoriant effects. They are very important in the control of severe pain of malignant disease but there are a number of adverse effects. Vomiting may occur but can be treated with cyclizine. Respiratory depression, smooth muscle spasm, hypotension and bradycardia may limit their use. Dependence occurs in some patients but this is not important in terminal disease. As the absorption after oral administration is variable, large doses of up to 60 mg may be needed. Increasing doses should be given in malignant disease until there is relief of pain, even if large doses such as 30—60 mg 4-hourly are required. As tolerance develops rapidly further increments may be required. A slow-release oral preparation of morphine sulphate has recently been formulated in which once- to twice-daily medication only is needed. This is a promising new preparation but more experience of its use is required. Morphia 10 mg i.m. or s.c. produces analgesia in 15—60 min, and i.v. administration gives earlier effects. Analgesia may last for 4—6 h but, if the duration is shorter, the doses should be repeated earlier. Another interesting development is the report of analgesia without significant adverse effects when given as an epidural injection (Behar *et al.*, 1979). The initial dose of heroin hydrochloride for parenteral use is 5—10 mg i.m. or s.c.

Methadone is more consistently effective than morphia when given orally. Dependence and tolerance develop more slowly. Because it has a long half-life, cumulation may occur, particularly in the frail and elderly. Methadone produces less vomiting than morphia and it is a cough-suppressant. As the euphoriant and sedative effects are less prominent than with morphia, it is less satisfactory in the control of pain in terminal disease. It is administered in 5—10 mg doses 4-hourly, s.c., i.m. or orally.

Pentazocine is of limited value in chronic pain. It lacks the euphoriant effect of morphia but it may induce withdrawal effects if added to regular opiate medication. The adverse effects, usually at higher doses, include nausea, vomiting, dizziness, sweating, hypotension, tachycardia, anxiety, nightmares or hallucinations. Local irritation may occur at the injection site. The dose of pentazocine is 25—100 mg orally, 3—4-hourly, or 30—60 mg i.m. 6—8-hourly. Nalorphine may be used for overdosage.

Pethidine is intermediate in potency between codeine and morphia but it is also unsatisfactory for the relief of chronic pain. It has a short duration of action of about 2 h only. There is a slight hypnotic effect, no important euphoriant action, and no cough-suppression. Some anticholinergic effects may occur with a dry mouth, blurred vision, but relatively little constipation. Hypotension and respiratory depression sometimes occur acutely. Dependence and tolerance may develop.

Naloxone is an opiate receptor blocker, now widely used in the research into enkephalins. It is used to reverse opiate-induced adverse effects, particularly respiratory depression in a dose of 0.4—1.2 mg i.v. An alternative method of treating opiate-induced respiratory depression is to use a respiratory stimulant, e.g. doxapram which probably acts by activation of carotid chemoreceptors to increase medullary respiratory drive. This may be given in 1—1.5 mg/kg doses i.v.

Other analgesics

Pholcodeine and dextromethorphan are used principally for cough-suppression as they do not have significant respiratory depression. Dipipanone combined with cyclizine (Diconal) may be a useful analgesic in ambulant patients with moderate pain. Oxycodone pectinate (Proladone) gives a longer duration of action at 8—14 h. Dextromoramide, oxycodone, phenazocine, and papaveretum are potent drugs but without proven superiority to heroin and morphia.

(c) Hypnotics

The loss of sleep produced by pain can be quite demoralising and it impairs the sufferer's capacity to cope with pain during the day. Hypnotics may therefore be useful. Nitrazepam 5—10 mg is satisfactory except for the long half-life causing a subtle dulling of intellect or unsteadiness of gait continuing into the following day. Tamazepam or chlormethiazole are shorter-acting alternatives. The older and now less fashionable hypnotics, choral hydrate or barbiturates, may also be considered in the patient with malignant disease.

(d) Phenothiazines

Chlorpromazine, fluphenazine or other phenothiazines may be used for their sedative, tranquillising and anti-emetic effects when pain is intractable in malignant disease. They are often unnecessary, however, with the use of appropriate analgesics. They potentiate the sedative but not the analgesic effects of narcotic drugs, and also potentiate hypnotics. The mild hypotensive, respiratory depressant and anticholinergic effects may sometimes present problems. An additional hazard is that sedation may turn to apathy, depression may be precipitated, impairing the patient's ability to cope with the illness. The starting dose of chlorpromazine is 25 mg, increasing to 100 mg q.i.d. if necessary.

(e) Butyrophenones

Haloperidol and droperidol have tranquillising effects, and may potentiate the analgesic but not the respiratory depressant effects of narcotic analgesics. They are used in combination with fentanyl or phenoperidine in neuroleptanalgesia but do not have an important place in the long-term control of pain.

(f) Benzodiazepines

Diazepam or chlordiazepoxide may be used in the patient in whom anxiety is unduly prominent but is not an alternative to the psychological support of patients and their relatives. Drowsiness is the most prominent adverse effect. Diazepam can be started at 2 mg t.i.d., but often 5–10 mg b.d. or t.i.d. is needed. It may also relieve muscle spasm. Chlordiazepoxide 10 mg t.i.d. has slightly less sedative effects than diazepam. Other benzodiazepine derivates such as oxazepam and lorazepam have not been shown to be more effective.

(g) Antidepressant drugs

The tricyclic antidepressants are most effective in patients with depression complicating chronic pain but are sometimes effective when depression is not overt, as in chronic facial pain. There is some evidence that tricyclics have effects on pain mechanisms separate from the antidepressant effects. Amitriptyline has a sedative action and is therefore useful if anxiety and agitation are prominent. In many patients a less sedative drug such as imipramine or nortriptyline may be preferred. If there is a risk of potentiating seizures nomifensine is preferable. Cardiac arrhythmias, hypotension, and anticholinergic adverse effects may be prominent. Tetracyclic drugs such as mianserin reduce these adverse effects and the toxicity of overdosage, but their use in chronic pain syndromes has not been evaluated. Glaucoma, cardiac disease and prostatic hypertrophy are contraindications to the use of tricyclic drugs. As all these drugs have long durations of action they may be administered once a day, preferably in the evening when the sedative effects are maximal. An explanation should be given that the improvement may not occur for many days after starting the drug or after an increment, and that sedation may be transient. A low initial dose is often needed such as 10–30 mg of amitriptyline nocte with weekly or fortnightly increments to 100 mg daily or more. The relationship between dose and plasma level is extremely variable with some patients metabolising the drug rapidly and others slowly. The relationship between plasma level and pain relief is uncertain.

(h) Monoamine oxidase inhibitors

Although these drugs may be effective in chronic pain syndromes they are seldom used now because drug interactions with analgesic drugs, sedatives and hypnotics make them more difficult to use than the tricyclic drugs, and they also carry the risk of hypertensive crises when tyramine-rich food is inadvertently taken.

(i) Carbamazepine

This is the drug of choice in trigeminal and glossopharyngeal neuralgias and it is also useful in painful paroxysmal disturbances in multiple sclerosis. Although less reliably effective it may be tried in other situations such as thalamic pain, post-herpetic neuralgia, neuralgia after sympathectomy, lightning pains of tabes dorsalis, and painful diabetic neuropathy. For adverse effects see Chapter 2. Phenytoin may also be used but it is usually less effective than carbamazepine.

(j) Placebos

Placebos improve symptoms in some pain syndromes such as migraine, but usually do not help in severe intractable pain. The placebo responses have long been considered a psychological phenomenon, but there has been recent evidence that they may be mediated *via* opiate receptors because their response is blocked with the opiate receptor blocker naloxone (Levine *et al.*, 1978).

4. Treatments that block conduction

Many attempts have been made to abolish pain either transiently or permanently by blocking or destroying conduction in peripheral nerves, nerve roots, or within the central nervous system. This variety in treatments is outlined here, but for detailed description of techniques of injection and the adverse effects the reader is referred to specialised publications (e.g. Swerdlow, 1977; Maher and Mehta, 1977).

Local analgesics

Local analgesic drugs, in dilute solution, block conduction in small fibres more than in large fibres but this differential block is difficult to achieve. In higher concentrations all fibres are blocked. Often the relief of pain may outlast the local analgesic effect. The accurate localisation of peripheral nerve injection sites may be aided with nerve-blocking aids which allow stimulation to identify the nerve prior to injection. Alternatively X-ray screening of the needle tip may help to localise deep injections. The two most useful local analgesic drugs are lignocaine and bupivacaine. Lignocaine may be administered as 1 or 2 per cent solutions, producing local anaesthetic effects for about 1 h. The total dose for a young, fit person should not exceed 7 mg/kg, but much less is used in the elderly and frail as sedative effects, convulsions or vascular collapse may occur. The duration of action is increased to about 2 h with adrenaline. Bupivacaine has a longer action, between 2 and 12 h, and is more potent than lignocaine. An 0.5 per cent solution is about equivalent to a 2 per cent solution of lignocaine and therefore 0.25 per cent solutions are suitable for most nerve blocks. The maximum dose for healthy adults should not exceed 2 mg/kg.

Neurolytic agents

Absolute alcohol is used for permanent nerve destruction but it may produce initial pain and local tenderness.

Phenol damages all fibre sizes after peripheral nerve or root injection but the destruction is greatest in small fibres. A 6 per cent solution can be used for peripheral nerve block but higher concentrations, up to 25 per cent in glycerol, may be used in intrathecal injections to produce permanent destruction of nerve roots. Another formulation for intrathecal injection is phenol in iodophendylate (Myodil) which allows its position to be seen on X-ray screening. A small initial injection of phenol may produce immediate analgesia or a warm sensation that helps to localise the site of the phenol before a larger amount is given to produce destructive changes.

Chlorocresol

This potent neurolytic agent is sometimes used for pain relief in malignant disease. It may be injected as 2 per cent concentration in glycerine intrathecally or 5 per cent for epidural block.

Injection sites

1. Musculoskeletal injections. Injections of local analgesic, e.g. at the facetal joints of the spine for chronic pain arising in the 'facetal syndrome', trigger points in the myofacial syndrome where major or minor trauma has produced pain, stiffness, limited movement and muscle spasm.

2. Somatic nerves. Somatic nerves, e.g. intercostal nerves for treatment of intercostal neuralgia where pain is prominent after surgery, fracture or tumour infiltration; the phrenic nerve in intractable hiccup; entrapment of a thoracic cutaneous nerve in the rectus sheath giving anterior abdominal pain; post-traumatic pain syndromes; occasional cases of entrapment of the lateral cutaneous nerve of the thigh; coccydynia, where pain follows major or repeated minor trauma in the coccygeal region. Some sites such as the maxillary nerve, mandibular nerve or Gasserian ganglion require considerable anatomical knowledge. Repeated local analgesic injections may be given. Sometimes it is wise to use an initial local analgesic injection and if temporary relief occurs then a more permanent destructive injection with a neurolytic agent is used.

3. Autonomic nervous system. Sympathetic blocks may relieve pain in a variety of syndromes, particularly where there is hyperpathia (Loh and Nathan, 1978). These include causalgia, Sudek's atrophy, the shoulder—hand syndrome, and phantom limb pain. If an initial local analgesic block is successful then a chemical or surgical sympathectomy should follow. Another form of sympathetic block uses a regional administration of guanethedine (Hannington-Kiff, 1979).

4. Extradural block. Local analgesic injection, sometimes in combination with steroids, may be used for severe abdominal pain where ventilatory depression is to be avoided, in a crushed chest, pain in malignant disease, and possibly for establishing whether intractable pain is organic or genuine. Several difficulties may arise. It may be difficult to check the level of injection initially, large volumes of analgesic may be required as it diffuses quite easily, and the technique is more difficult than the intradural blocks. Special needles are recommended. It is possible to give continuous analgesic infusion *via* a catheter for several days. The hazards of the technique are inadvertent dural puncture, intravascular injection, hypotension, and transient paralysis (very occasional permanent weakness).

5. Intrathecal block. Intractable pain in malignant disease and severe painful spasm may be treated with phenol. Very careful positioning of the patient is needed to limit the destruction to the desired nerve roots. As sphincter disturbances are major risks after lumbar injection many physicians prefer to restrict the use of intrathecal phenol to patients that have already lost bladder function, e.g. in multiple sclerosis with paraplegia. Weakness and sensory loss in the affected root distribution are to be expected. The duration of pain relief is variable. It may last for days, weeks, months or it may be permanent. Intrathecal phenol has also been used in the thoracic and cervical regions but the technique requires considerable skill.

6. *Hypertonic saline and CSF barbotage.* These rather crude techniques are reported, perhaps surprisingly, to relieve pain in patients with malignant disease and to have relatively minor adverse effects. Cold hypertonic saline injected into the subarachnoid space may relieve pain for up to 3 months but it requires to be done under general anaesthesia (Hitchcock and Prandini, 1973). In CSF barbotage, the alternate removal and injection of 10 ml CSF, at normal temperature or cooled, may relieve pain but the results were reported in a small series only (Lloyd *et al.*, 1972).

Surgical procedures

1. Peripheral nerve section

Although division of peripheral nerves in chronic pain is superficially attractive the results are often unsatisfactory. It causes permanent anaesthesia, sometimes weakness, and is often ineffective. Furthermore, a nerve section may be complicated by the development of a neuroma at the cut end, producing dysaesthesiae and pain.

2. Rhizotomy

Rhizotomy avoids the motor complications of peripheral nerve section, but may be complicated by proprioceptive defects, trophic changes and skin ulcers. It is therefore not a satisfactory procedure for pain in the limbs but may be used for pain in the trunk. Rhizotomy must include division of the roots in the segments above and below the root with pain. The most satisfactory selective nerve root section is in the treatment of trigeminal neuralgia as the maxillary or mandibular roots can be selectively divided, preserving the ophthalmic division, and avoiding the hazard of corneal ulceration.

3. Cordotomy

An anterolateral cordotomy divides the lateral spinothalamic pathways. Although pain is abolished initially in about 70 per cent of patients it returns within 18 months, accompanied by unpleasant dysaesthesiae. Cordotomy may therefore be considered for the relief of intractable pain from malignant disease where the life-expectancy is short, but it is not satisfactory for patients with pain of a benign aetiology. The operation may be done as an open procedure or by percutaneous cervical cordotomy. The main immediate hazard is that the lesion may interrupt the adjacent corticospinal pathways producing hemiparesis. Bilateral cordotomy carries an additional risk of sphincter disturbance, impotence, and impaired blood pressure control.

4. Lesions at intracranial sites

Intracranial stereotactic procedures are occasionally used to relieve pain. Lateral mesencephalic tractotomy may be effective, but carries the risk of diplopia, refractory dysaesthesia, and hemiparesis. Trigeminal tractotomy is also rather unsatisfactory. Thalamotomies have been used with mixed success. The best results are with lesions in both medial and lateral nuclear groups, but such multi-staged procedures have few indications.

Stimulation techniques in pain relief

1. Transcutaneous nerve stimulation

In this technique low-intensity electrical stimulation is given by large surface electrodes in or near the affected region. It should be of such a low stimulus strength that the patient is just aware of it. Most equipment permits the control of the stimulus duration, frequency and intensity. An initial response rate of 20—25 per cent of patients may occur but the success rate subsequently falls considerably and the long-term results are poor. As the technique is without hazard and the responders cannot be predicted, there is a place for a therapeutic trial in chronic pain, including the usually refractory groups of post-herpetic and post-traumatic neuralgias.

2. Peripheral nerve stimulation

These techniques are more invasive as they use implanted electrodes. Some success has been reported with pain arising from peripheral nerve injury, but experience has not been extensive.

3. Acupuncture

The mechanism is uncertain but it could involve the enkephalin systems in the CNS. Its use as an analgesic for surgery is widely publicised but its role in the long-term relief of chronic pain is unclear. Single or multiple needles may be used either twisted, with vibration, with low-intensity electrical stimulation, and even, more fashionably, with lasers.

4. Dorsal column stimulation

Electrodes are positioned over the dorsal columns of the spinal cord either extradurally by a percutaneous technique or in the subarachnoid space. As the complication rate, particularly CSF leak, is higher with the latter technique, extradural placement of the electrodes is usually preferable. Stimulation is *via* a subcutaneous radiotelemetric receiver, activated by an external transmitter. Because of the expense of stimulators and the long-term problems of electrode movement, equipment failure, arachnoiditis, and infection dorsal column stimulation has a limited place in pain relief.

5. Periaqueductal and periventricular grey matter

Pain relief occurs with stimulation of the periventricular grey matter deep to the third ventricle, and in the periaqueductal region. These findings are of considerable theoretical interest as the pain relief may arise from activation of the descending inhibitory pathways to the cord, and the projection of the reticular formation to the cortex. They are, however, of limited general application.

Pituitary neuroadenolysis. Destruction of the pituitary gland by ethanol injection into the pituitary fossa sometimes reduces pain in patients with hormone-dependent tumours of the breast, prostate, thyroid gland or endometrium. Improvement has also been reported in other tumours not traditionally considered as hormone-dependent (Moricca, 1977). A relatively non-invasive technique, using a trans-nasal, trans-sphenoidal injection of alcohol, is used. Hypothalamic damage with coma, hyperphagia, and hypothermia may occur. Other complications include headache, CSF rhinorrhoea, meningitis, and hypopituitarism. The advantage of the technique is that relief of diffuse or multiple pains may be achieved without either multiple regional in-jection, or the use of potent drugs. The pain relief may last in some patients months or years, but patients with only transient relief may have a repeat alcohol injection. The mechanism is intriguing but poorly understood.

CLINICAL PROBLEMS

Trigeminal neuralgia

Carbamazepine is the treatment of choice but as some elderly patients tolerate it poorly it should be started in a low dose. Phenytoin or clonazepam are only occasionally helpful. About 20 per cent of patients do not have adequate pain relief from carbamazepine 200–1000 mg daily and require a nerve block with alcohol or a rhizotomy. An alternative to an open selective nerve root section is the use of radiofrequency thermocoagulation under neuroleptanalgesia. This procedure has the advantage that touch is preserved, and as the morbidity is low, it is suitable for the frail and elderly (Sengupta and Stunden, 1977).

Post-herpetic neuralgia

This condition is sometimes distressingly resistant to treatment. Simple analgesics are usually ineffective, and there is a tendency to give progressively more potent analgesics. Where there are paroxysmal components to the pain, carbamazepine may be helpful but it is seldom useful for the background of continuous pain. Tricyclic drugs occasionally reduce the pain. Simple non-invasive techniques are rather disappointing but may be tried — local ethylchloride spray, or percussion with a mechanical vibrator. Transcutaneous nerve stimulation relieves pain in some patients, including small numbers with total relief, and the analgesia can persist after stopping stimulation (Nathan and Wall, 1974). In the majority it is ineffective. Nerve and root section is unsatisfactory. A hypnotic is indicated when sleep is disturbed.

It is impossible to predict which patient with acute herpes zoster will develop post-herpetic neuralgia. Amantadine is of doubtful value in preventing the neuralgia.

Local idoxyuridine may reduce the local ocular complications of herpes zoster infection but not the neuralgia. Sympathectomy within the first 6 months is reported to reduce the prevalence and severity of subsequent post-herpetic neuralgia but further experience is required.

Multiple sclerosis

Paroxysmal pain in multiple sclerosis is best treated with carbamazepine. Painful muscle spasm is reduced with spasmolytic drugs (*see* Chapter 7), and occasionally intrathecal phenol is needed.

Causalgia

This persistent, often distressing, pain after nerve trauma is difficult to treat. Simple analgesics or transcutaneous nerve stimulation are usually unsatisfactory, and pain is likely to recur after section of the affected nerve. Sympathectomy is the technique most likely to be helpful. An alternative to local analgesic block is the use of guanethidine injected i.v. after application of a tourniquet (Hannington-Kiff, 1979).

Persistent benign pain syndromes

These may be treated with the techniques already discussed, mild analgesics, carbamazepine, transcutaneous stimulation, acupuncture, and hypnotherapy, psychotherapy and behaviour therapy are sometimes helpful. Invasive stimulation techniques such as stimulation of the dorsal column or the mesencephalon require careful assessment in specialised units. The temptation to use destructive central lesions such as cordotomy should be avoided as the relief is often transient.

Pain in malignant disease

The aim should be to relieve pain, maintain mental clarity, optimism and mobility for as long as possible. Each pain should be assessed carefully. Smooth muscle spasm is best treated with a spasmolytic drug such as probanthine. Nerve entrapment can be helped with steroids or local analgesic injections. The adverse effects of analgesic drugs must be considered; in particular, weakness and lethargy leading to immobility and dehydration. The choice of analgesic drugs and physical treatment should be based on the principles discussed earlier. Pituitary adenolysis may be considered in the patient with multiple or intractable pain.

HEADACHE

This section is concerned with chronic or recurrent disorders in which headache is the main or the only symptom. Migraine and tension headaches are the commonest of these disorders but atypical facial pain, trigeminal neuralgia, temporomandibular arthropathy and cervical spondylosis are also discussed. The small number of patients with cough or exertional headache, a disorder of obscure but benign mechanisms, require explanation and reassurance. It should be recognised, in assessing patients with headache, that hypertension causes headaches only when severe, usually with a diastolic pressure exceeding 120 mmHg. Another common misinterpretation is the attribution of headaches to refractive errors.

Migraine

Pathogenesis

Many ideas have been proposed to explain migraine but a coherent account has not yet emerged. The longest-established hypothesis is that there is an initial period of vasoconstriction, accompanied by reduced cerebral blood flow, in which focal ischaemic symptoms may occur. This is followed by vasodilatation of external carotid arteries, when the headache occurs. This is an inadequate explanation and other mechanisms are involved. An origin in the nociceptive endings in the meningeal vessels has been postulated (Blau, 1978). Another hypothesis suggests release from the trigeminal nerve of a vasoactive substance-P and 5-hydroxytryptamine (5-HT) (Moskowitz *et al.*, 1979). A central origin has been proposed (Sicuteri, 1976). The mechanisms underlying these vascular and neural changes are complex. Vasoactive amines affect vasomotor function, permeability, and pain. The best-documented of these complex changes is 5-HT which is released from platelets during an attack, the plasma level falls, and the excretion of its metabolites increases. The 5-HT may act by producing vasoconstriction of the external carotid arteries. Other biochemical changes occur before, during and after migraine. High plasma noradrenaline has been reported in the hours prior to migraine which occurs on wakening. The local release of bradykinin, other kinins and histamine have also been implicated in migraine. The activity of monoamine oxidase, particularly for phenylethylamine metabolism, is reduced during migraine (Sandler *et al.*, 1974). Platelet aggregation is increased during the attack.

Alterations in sodium and water retention, ammonia, glucose and free fatty acid metabolism have been reported but are of uncertain significance. Patients may describe periods of euphoria, increased appetite, and drowsiness before the attack itself, suggesting a central, probably hypothalamic, disturbance. In view of all these metabolic changes it is not surprising that many drugs have been tried, predominantly those affecting monoamine metabolism or receptor function, and that the success has been mixed.

Management

Many patients cope well with their migraine without the aid of physicians, using simple analgesics as necessary. Patients may seek advice with frequent severe common migraine in which unilateral throbbing headache may be accompanied by nausea and photophobia. Classical migraine occurs less frequently than common migraine but it produces more anxiety initially as visual symptoms may occur, or the attack may be accompanied by a wide range of other features including hemiplegia, dysphasia and sensory symptoms. Complicated migraine includes patients with very prolonged focal features, severe vertebrobasilar ischaemia, confusion, coma, ophthalmoplegia, or even infarction. Patients presenting with complicated migraine may require careful investigation to exclude other disorders.

General measures

A careful discussion is needed in which possible initiating or potentiating factors are considered with a view to avoiding them if possible. Stress is commonly a factor but the stereotype of a migraine personality with rigid, perfectionist, striving attitudes is not generally applicable. Paradoxically, relaxation after stress may trigger attacks. If there are attitudes or factors in the environment that may be altered, the physician should encourage this. Depression may increase the liability to attacks, and requires treatment.

Dietary precipitants are found in only a small proportion of patients and the commonest are coffee, chocolate, monosodium glutamate, and alcohol. A trial period of withdrawal from possible precipitants for a few weeks may be followed by reintroduction of each possible precipitant. Studies of dietary precipitants such as tyramine (in cheese) and phenylethylamine (in chocolate) have not yielded consistent results. These precipitants probably trigger a series of vasomotor changes but should not be regarded as an allergy as there is no evidence that they involve immune mechanisms. Another avoidable trigger is hypoglycaemia.

Menstrual migraine is common but may be difficult to abolish. The results of treatment of fluid retention with a mild diuretic a few days before the onset of periods, or the use of a progestagen, are often unsatisfactory. The effects of oral contraceptives on migraine are varied and the mechanisms of the changes obscure. In many patients migraine has preceded the use of oral contraceptives and remains unaltered by them, while in others the migraine starts after regularly taking oral contraceptives for months or years. There is no indication for withdrawal of the oral contraceptives in these groups. Some patients experience an increase in headache with oral contraceptives. If the pattern of the headache changes, particularly with the development of visual or other focal symptoms, then oral contraceptives should be withdrawn because of the risk of migrainous infarction. The risk is impossible to measure for there has been no researcher so bold or foolish to study this in a prospective manner.

If attacks are triggered by bright lights then dark glasses may be helpful. In the small group of patients with attacks triggered on sexual intercourse, drugs may be preferred to abstinence. Sport which triggers recurrent or severe migraine, e.g. footballer's migraine, may have to be stopped.

Success has been claimed in small groups of selected patients using techniques which enhance relaxation (Warner and Lance, 1975), hypnosis, and biofeedback techniques (Medina *et al.*, 1976). These techniques are difficult to apply widely but may have a place in centres with the necessary skills in selected patients with frequent stress-related migraine attacks.

Treatment of the acute attack

Many patients prefer to retire to a quiet, darkened room during the attack. Aspirin 300—600 mg or paracetamol 0.5—1 g may be taken at the start of the headache. Metoclopramide 10 mg, cyclizine or prochlorperazine may be useful if nausea and vomiting occur. Metoclopramide enhances gastric emptying and the absorption of analgesic drugs. Recently, preparations have been marketed combining aspirin or paracetamol with metoclopramide. Occasionally unpleasant severe dystonic reactions are produced by metoclopramide.

Ergotamine tartrate has been used for many years. It is an alkaloid with direct vasoconstrictor actions on extracranial vessels. There is additional evidence that it may have dual effects, constricting dilated vessels and dilating vasoconstricted ones, and this may account for the absence of exacerbation of visual and other focal symptoms in classical migraine. Despite the drug's long use in migraine, controlled trials have been few and conflicting in their results. As some patients respond to ergotamine given at the start of a headache, it may be tried in patients with attacks refractory to simple analgesics. Oral administration produces unreliable results because of the varied rates of absorption and the occurrence of vomiting. It may be given orally together with an anti-emetic, e.g. cyclizine. Caffeine is added to some proprietary preparations with the aim of enhancing absorption. Sublingual or rectal administration are alternative routes. An inhaler may be used but the patient has to be entirely reliable because it is very easy to produce overdosage. Parenteral ergotamine is rarely needed. The oral dose of ergotamine tartrate is 0.5—2 mg initially, and this may be repeated in 30—45 min. If the patient does not respond to this dose, he or she is unlikely to respond to higher doses. Therefore repeated doses up to the manufacturer's recommended limits of 6 mg daily and 10 mg weekly are to be avoided. The patients taking larger doses or frequent ergotamine are better tried on alternative drugs for they may suffer intoxication with a syndrome of recurrent headaches, nausea and malaise which only disappears on withdrawal of ergotamine. If necessary the patient should be admitted to hospital for the ergotamine withdrawal. Because ergotamine has vasoconstrictor effects, it should be avoided in patients with ischaemic heart disease, peripheral vascular disease, and in pregnancy, and should also be avoided in patients with hepatic and renal insufficiency.

Isometheptene is an alternative to ergotamine for the acute headache. It is formulated in a 65 mg dose with dichloralphenazone 100 mg and paracetamol 325 mg (Midrid). Two tablets are taken initially, then one each hour up to a maximum of five in 12 h.

In prolonged intractable migraine (status migrainosis) prednisolone 40–60 mg daily for 3 days may be effective. The steroid is then gradually withdrawn on subsequent days.

Prophylactic drugs

When a patient has frequent migraine attacks which are not satisfactorily controlled by simple analgesic drugs or ergotamine a prophylactic drug is indicated. The variety of drugs reported to have value in the prophylaxis of migraine reflects their relative ineffectiveness. As the placebo response is high, in many drug trials between 30 and 60 per cent, only careful controlled trials are acceptable. The 5-HT blockers, methysergide, pizotifen, and cyproheptadine are moderately successful prophylactic drugs.

Methysergide (Deseril) is the longest-established effective prophylactic drug but its use is limited by a variety of adverse effects including gastrointestinal symptoms, light-headedness and insomnia. The most important side-effect is the risk of retroperitoneal and mediastinal fibrosis with continued use. Therefore, it should be restricted to refractory migraine and it should be given intermittently. The safe limits are not clearly known but administration for 2–3 months followed by 2 months without methysergide prevents the irreversible fibrosis. The usual dose is 3–6 mg daily, starting in a low dose of 1 mg daily, with gradual increments, if necessary, in subsequent weeks.

Pizotifen (Sanomigran) is better than placebo in controlled trials and does not cause retroperitoneal fibrosis with prolonged treatment. Weight-gain due to appetite stimulation is a common adverse effect.

Dizziness, drowsiness and tingling of the extremities may also occur. The starting dose is 0.5 mg t.i.d., but if the migraine is not controlled on this dose it should be increased to 1 mg t.i.d.

Cyproheptadine (Periactin) is an alternative prophylactic drug, less effective than methysergide, with some sedative side-effects and a tendency to produce weight-gain, but it does not produce retroperitoneal fibrosis. The dose is 4—8 mg daily, starting in a low dose of 2 mg b.d.

Propranolol, the β-blocker, has been found to significantly reduce the frequency and severity of attacks in a number of trials. Small doses, e.g. 10 mg t.i.d., may occasionally be effective but commonly a higher dose of 80—160 mg daily is required. It may be more effective in patients with prominent anxiety. It is contraindicated in asthma and cardiac failure. Bradycardia, hypotension, cardiac failure, bronchoconstriction, nausea and vomiting, occasional bowel disturbances and depression are possible adverse effects. Most patients with migraine tolerate it well. Withdrawal should be gradual. Other β-blockers such as oxyprenolol and pindolol have not been studied adequately but may well differ in their effectiveness from propranolol.

Amitriptyline is probably comparable to propranolol and almost as effective as methysergide. Its action in the prevention of migraine appears to be separable from the effects against depression (Couch and Hassanein, 1979). Surprisingly, it is reported to be less effective in patients with associated depression. The dosage range is 25—100 mg daily, starting at 25 mg nocte, with increments of 25 mg every 1—2 weeks until there is control or adverse effects. As trials have not included plasma levels the relationship between the plasma level and response is unknown. The adverse effects are drowsiness, cardiac arrhythmias, an increased risk of seizures, and anticholinergic effects such as dry mouth, constipation and glaucoma. The effectiveness of less sedative tricyclic drugs such as nortriptyline, and of tetracyclic drugs, has yet to be established.

Aspirin 650 mg b.d. has been reported to reduce the frequency of headaches in some patients in a very small study of 12 patients (O'Neill and Mann, 1978).

Clonidine (Dixarit) has been disappointing. The initial claims for benefit in doses of 50—100 μg daily have not been supported by controlled trials although some patients appear to have some benefit.

Migrainous neuralgia (cluster headache)

The clusters of intense, distressing frontal and facial pain of migrainous neuralgia must be clearly distinguished from trigeminal neuralgia, dental pain, sinusitis, etc. for the treatment is different. The mechanisms have been less extensively studied than in migraine but there is evidence implicating changes in 5-HT and platelets during the attacks. There are usually no identifiable environmental stimuli except that some patients may have a seasonal occurrence, and prophylactic treatment can be started at these times.

The prophylactic drugs such as pizotifen or methysergide may be used. If the clusters have a predictable duration the drug should be withdrawn after this. If the duration is variable the drug should be withdrawn after an arbitrary period such as 1 month, and recommenced if there are further episodes.

Ergotamine tartrate has been used for many years. It may be given regularly for the duration of the cluster, e.g. 0.5–1 mg orally at night and in the morning. If it is ineffective by this route, it may be administered as 0.5 mg s.c. If successful the patient may be taught to administer the drug himself. Steroids may be used in intractable cases (Couch and Hassanein, 1979).

Lithium carbonate 250 mg t.i.d. is helpful in clusters of migrainous neuralgia, and in the chronic variants.

Tension headache

The mechanisms producing the chronic or recurrent pain of tension headache or muscle contraction headache are both psychogenic and physical. The patients' anxieties, frustration, or depression may be clearly recognised in many patients; other patients deny such mechanisms. Sometimes the fear that the cause of the headache might be an undiagnosed tumour or threatened cerebral haemorrhage is not verbalised until tactfully discussed by the physician.

The physical changes that accompany the headaches are a background of continuous muscle contraction in the scalp, at times extending also to the neck and the masseters. Local tenderness or trigger points may be present. There are changes in local blood flow, sometimes with reduction in muscle perfusion, sometimes with increased flow, and these may be the basis for the throbbing component which is sometimes felt.

Many mildly affected patients clearly recognise the role of tension and do not seek medical aid. In contrast the chronic sufferer may complain of continuous intractable headache. Careful assessment of the patient's home, work, social background, and fears about the cause of the headache is needed. The treatment may have various components.

(1) Explain and reassure. Careful examination, explanation and discussion may be sufficient.

(2) Manipulate the stress-producing situations in the environment if possible. This might involve changes in the patient's job or the home.

(3) Encourage techniques in relaxation. The choice depends on the patient's preferences and the availability of particular skills. Yoga, biofeedback, and hypnosis have all been used.

(4) Drug therapy. Mild analgesics such as aspirin and paracetamol may be helpful. Anxiolytic drugs are generally disappointing. They may relieve anxiety in the short term and reduce muscle tone but do not provide long-term solutions, and may exacerbate problems by impairing the patient's ability to cope with anxiety. Amitriptyline may help and is superior to simple analgesics, benzodiazepines, and treatments which alter blood flow (Lance and Curran, 1964).

(5) Psychotherapy. The good physician provides simple psychotherapy during the interview but usually cannot provide the detailed psychological support that a few disturbed patients require. For these psychiatric help is indicated.

Atypical facial pain

This syndrome is of uncertain aetiology but may respond to tricyclic drugs although depression may not be overt. Occasionally carbamazepine is beneficial. Tranquillisers and mild or moderate analgesics are usually unsatisfactory. These patients may be fearful that they may have an unrecognised neoplasm or other serious condition. These fears are best discussed and firm reassurance given.

Temporomandibular arthropathy

Temporomandibular arthropathy (Costen's syndrome) requires dental treatment with prostheses to alter the bite.

Cervical spondylosis

Cervical spondylosis and soft tissue injury in the upper cervical regions may produce severe or recurrent pain in the neck, mastoid and occipital regions. Occasionally, these pains radiate to the temporal and even to the frontal regions. Various treatments have been applied. Some patients improve spontaneously while others are helped by a cervical collar which reduces inadvertent neck movements and the traction on affected nerves. The value of manipulation or traction is unclear but undoubtedly some patients are improved. The infiltration of local analgesic into supporting ligaments and tendon insertions in the cervical region may provide relief (Blumenthal, 1974).

Post-traumatic syndrome (post-concussional)

This syndrome occurs after a minor head injury. Recurrent headaches develop and there may be bouts of dizziness, transient visual disturbances, difficulty in concentration, irritability and nervousness. It is likely that these have an organic basis although there have been arguments that they are all psychological. The symptoms eventually settle although it may take weeks, months, or even years. Reassurance and explanation are needed. Simple analgesics may help the headaches. Prochlorperazine (Stemetil) may help if vertigo is prominent.

REFERENCES

Behar, M, Magora, F, Olshwang, D and Davidson, J T (1979) Epidural morphine in the treatment of pain. *Lancet*, **1**, 527–529.

Blau, J N (1978) Migraine: A vasomotor instability of the meningeal circulation. *Lancet*, **2**, 1136–1139.

Blumenthal, L S (1974) Injury to the cervical spine as a cause of headache. *Postgraduate Medicine*, **56**, 147–153.

Couch, J R and Ziegler, D K (1978) Prednisolone therapy for cluster headaches. *Headache*, **18**, 219–221.

Couch, J R and Hassanein, R S (1979) Amitriptyline in migraine prophylaxis. *Archives of Neurology*, **36**, 695–699.

Hannington-Kiff, J G (1979) Relief of causalgia in limbs by regional intravenous guanethidine. *British Medical Journal*, **2**, 367–368.

Hitchcock, E and Prandini, M N (1973) Hypertonic saline in management of intractable pain. *Lancet*, **1**, 310–312.

Lance, J W and Curran, D A (1964) Treatment of chronic tension headache. *Lancet*, **1**, 1236–1239.

Levine, J D, Gordon, N C and Fields, H L (1978) The mechanism of placebo analgesia. *Lancet*, **2**, 654–657.

Lloyd, J W, Hughes, J T and Davies-Jones, G A B (1972) Relief of severe intractable pain by barbotage of cerebrospinal fluid. *Lancet*, **1**, 354–355.

Loh, L and Nathan, P W (1978) Painful peripheral states and sympathetic blocks. *Journal of Neurology, Neurosurgery and Psychiatry*, **41**, 664–671.

Maher, R and Mehta, M (1977) Spinal (intradural) and extradural analgesia. In: *Persistent Pain: Modern Methods of Treatment*, vol. I, pp. 61–99. (Ed) S Lipton. Academic Press, London; Grune & Stratton, New York.

Medina, J L. Diamond, S and Franklin, M A (1976) Biofeedback therapy for migraine. *Headache*, **16**, 115—118.

Moricca, G (1977) Pituitary neuroadenolysis in the treatment of intractable pain from cancer. In: *Persistent Pain: Modern Methods of Treatment*, vol. I, pp. 149—173. (Ed) S. Lipton. Academic Press, London; Grune & Stratton, New York.

Moskowitz, M A, Reinhard J F, Romero, J, Melamed, E and Pettibone, D J (1979) Neurotransmitter and the fifth cranial nerve: is there a relation to the headache phase of migraine? *Lancet*, **2**, 883—885.

Nathan, P W and Wall, P D (1974) Treatment of post-herpetic neuralgia by prolonged electric stimulation. *British Medical Journal*, **3**, 645—647.

O'Neill, B P and Mann, J D (1978) Aspirin prophylaxis in migraine. *Lancet*, **2**, 1179—1181.

Sandler, M, Youdim, M B H and Hanington, E (1974) A phenylethylamine oxidising defect in migraine. *Nature*, **250**, 335—337.

Sengupta, R P and Stunden, R J (1977) Radiofrequency thermocoagulation of Gasserian ganglion and its rootlets for trigeminal neuralgia. *British Medical Journal*, **1**, 142—143.

Sicuteri, F (1976) Migraine: a central biochemical dysnocioception. *Headache*, **16**, 145—159.

Swerdlow, M (1977) Peripheral nerve blocking in the relief of pain. In: *Persistent Pain: Modern Methods of Treatment*, vol. I, pp. 207—235. (Ed) S Lipton. Academic Press, London; Grune & Stratton, New York.

Warner, G and Lance, L W (1975) Relaxation therapy in migraine and chronic tension headache. *The Medical Journal of Australia*, **1**, 298—301.

CHAPTER SEVEN

Demyelinating Disorders

Although the myelin sheath of nerve fibres both in the peripheral and central nervous systems is affected in a wide variety of neurological disorders demyelination of the white matter of the central nervous system with relative preservation of axons is the predominant feature in the pathology of the primary demyelinating diseases. This group of disorders includes multiple sclerosis, acute disseminated encephalomyelitis, neuromyelitis optica (Devic's disease) and Schilder's disease. Multiple sclerosis is a common disorder with a prevalence in northern Europe in excess of 50/100,000. Acute disseminated encephalomyelitis is a rare complication of certain virus infections, such as measles and chicken pox, and vaccination. Pathologically it resembles experimental allergic encephalomyelitis in animals and probably represents an allergic reaction of the nervous system to a virus infection. Neuromyelitis optica is a rare disorder which pathologically resembles multiple sclerosis but in its natural history has a greater similarity to acute disseminated encephalomyelitis. Schilder's disease is a rare disorder of childhood in which there is extensive demyelination of the cerebral hemispheres and its precise relationship to multiple sclerosis on the one hand and the leucodystrophies on the other is uncertain.

MULTIPLE SCLEROSIS

The aetiology of this disease is still imperfectly understood but there is now a substantial body of evidence that one factor may be exposure to a virus infection in childhood, which may perhaps persist in the nervous system in certain individuals with a genetically determined abnormality in the immune system. Evidence for a genetic susceptibility arises from the increased incidence of multiple sclerosis in relatives of patients and the association of the disease with patients' HLA tissue type antigens. In addition the similarity of the morbid anatomy to that of experimental allergic encephalomyelitis and the presence of abnormal immuno-globulins in the CSF provide suggestive evidence for an abnormality in the immune system. The geographical distribution of the disease is of particular interest. In both northern and southern hemispheres it is more prevalent in regions remote from the equator but when areas are studied which have a high immigrant population, such as Israel and South Africa, it would appear that the risk to any individual is dependent on where the individual has spent the early years of life. This would suggest an exogenous factor present in childhood. No viral agent has been identified but there are many reports of elevated titres of measles and other virus agents in patients with multiple sclerosis (Brody *et al.*, 1972) and there have been a number of reports providing evidence for a transmissible agent in tissues of patients with multiple sclerosis (Field, 1966; Carp *et al.*, 1972). There is also evidence that there may be an abnormality in fatty acid metabolism in multiple sclerosis. Thus the white matter of the brains of patients with multiple sclerosis has been found to contain less unsaturated fatty acid than controls and lowered concentrations of linoleic acid have also been found in the serum of multiple sclerosis patients (Thompson, 1975). This could be one factor in an abnormality of immune mechanisms since polyunsaturated fatty acids may inhibit the lymphocyte immune response (Mertin and Caspary, 1975).

Pathology and prognosis

Naked eye examination of the nervous system in multiple sclerosis shows the presence of plaques of demyelination scattered throughout the white matter of the brain and spinal cord. Microscopically, there is loss of myelin and in the acute state of the illness there is a lymphocytic reaction surrounding the blood vessels with glial proliferation and loss of oligodendrocytes. Histochemically there is loss of myelin basic protein with an excess of proteolytic enzymes. Immunofluorescence techniques have demonstrated both immunoglobulin and complement within the plaques.

There is great variation in the natural history of multiple sclerosis and it is difficult to assess the prognosis for the individual patient. In some instances the illness will start acutely at a young age and will run a rapidly progressive course with a fatal outcome in a few years. In other patients the disease has a very benign course with long survival and little disability after 20 or 30 years. The average life-expectancy is of the order of 20 years. The age of onset is commonly in the third or fourth decades and progression may take the form of remissions and relapses, the patient eventually becoming chairbound and bedridden, death eventually occurring from intercurrent infection particularly of the urinary tract. In the later stages mental changes may occur and may take the form of euphoria, depression or a falling-off of intellectual capacities. If the first symptom is one of optic neuritis the development of further symptoms may be delayed for many years and a substantial number of patients who have optic neuritis never develop other symptoms of multiple sclerosis. A progressive form of the illness with mainly spinal symptoms and with little tendency to remission not infrequently develops when the disease first presents in later life in patients over the age of 40.

It must be recognised that although specific therapy for the disease falls far short of what is desirable there is much that can be done to relieve individual symptoms and to treat complications.

The acute attack – the use of steroids

Acute exacerbations of multiple sclerosis have a tendency to recover spontaneously so that the assessment of the value of any form of therapy is difficult and requires carefully controlled studies. General measures are frequently helpful and many will benefit if they are admitted to hospital in the acute stage. Here initial rest with passive movements to paralysed and spastic limbs may be followed by mobilisation with active physiotherapy as the condition improves. It is important to recognise and treat any intercurrent infection, particularly of the urinary tract. A number of controlled studies have appeared to indicate that corticotrophin is of value in shortening the duration of an acute relapse (Miller *et al.*, 1961; Rose *et al.*, 1970). Although the acute episode may resolve more quickly in the treated patients it is less certain whether the treatment of relapses in this way has any significant effect on the long-term status of the patient (Bowden *et al.*, 1974). Why ACTH should be effective is uncertain. The effect is probably too rapid for it to be due to immunosuppression and one possibility is that it is acting simply by reducing oedema which could clearly be an important mechanism in the response to treatment of optic neuritis. Tourtellotte (1975) has suggested that the action of ACTH and steroids is through an anti-inflammatory effect, and they have provided data to indicate that in an exacerbation of multiple sclerosis the synthesis of IgG in the central nervous system is decreased by ACTH and steroids. If ACTH is given it may be started in a dose of 80 units daily which can be gradually reduced and eventually discontinued after 4–6 weeks but shorter courses may be appropriate with mild relapses. There are many hazards in the long-term administration of corticotrophin or steroids. In addition to hypersensitivity reactions they may aggravate infection, hypertension or diabetes and give rise to haemorrhage in patients with peptic ulceration, and in some subjects will provoke psychotic reactions. They generally cause retention of sodium and loss of potassium and over the long term may lead to osteoporosis and cataract. The short-term administration is relatively safe provided contraindications are avoided, but it may sometimes be advisable to give medication with antacids and also diuretics if oedema is present. It is useful when a course of corticotrophin is started to confirm that the preparation is active by checking the plasma cortisol levels of the patient before and after therapy is started. Long-term therapy with corticotrophin appears to be of no value (Millar *et al.*, 1967). In the early studies of ACTH in the treatment of acute exacerbations it was suggested that corticotrophin was more effective than prednisone and the idea was put forward that it might act by promoting the release of other substances in addition to cortisone from the adrenal cortex. There is, however, no definite evidence of this, and oral steroids can be used (Edie and Tyrer, 1980).

Prevention of relapses — immunosuppressive drugs and diet

Long-term treatment with steroids has been found to be ineffective in preventing relapses and likewise no benefit has been found with azathioprine given long-term in low dosage (Swinburn and Liversedge, 1973). On the other hand Rosen (1979) has found that azathioprine given daily over a period of years to a group of patients with non-remitting multiple sclerosis appeared to slow the progress of the disease. More radical methods of immunosuppression include the use of steroids along with azathioprine and antilymphocytic globulin, and some reduction in relapse rate has been claimed for this therapy which is still, however, in the experimental stage (Lance *et al.*, 1975). A different approach to immunological therapy has been to administer dialysable transfer factor obtained from human peripheral blood leucocytes, but therapeutic trials of this therapy have shown little benefit (Fog *et al.*, 1975; Zabriskie *et al.*, 1975; Behan *et al.*, 1976). The production of a relapsing form of experimental encephalomyelitis — by the injection of purified myelin fraction with Freund's adjuvant in the guinea pig — which closely resembles human multiple sclerosis (Lassmann and Wisniewski, 1979) gives hope that eventually the disease could be suppressed by desensitisation with myelin basic protein given without adjuvant, or more safely by means of synthetic non-encephalitic peptides (Hallpike, 1980).

The value of unsaturated fatty acids such as linoleic acid was studied by Millar and a group of co-workers in 1973 who found in a double-blind controlled trial that linoleic acid taken in the form of 30 ml of sunflower-seed oil emulsion per day had some effect in reducing the frequency and severity of relapses; a reduction in severity of relapses has also been reported by Bates *et al.* (1978). Field and Joyce (1979) suggest that γ-linolenate may benefit patients with early disease but controlled observations are needed to confirm this. Other dietary measures that have been advocated include a gluten-free diet. This theory is based on the suggestion that areas of high prevalence of multiple sclerosis correspond with areas of high wheat consumption (Shatin, 1964) but so far pilot studies of this therapy have not confirmed its value (Liversedge, 1975). In general it is advisable that patients with multiple sclerosis should not put on excessive weight, and if sunflower-seed oil is taken some restriction of caloric intake from other foods is indicated. At the present time, the treatment of the chronic relapsing or slowly progressive case of multiple sclerosis remains unsatisfactory. No regime of immunosuppressive steroid therapy has been shown to be of definite value in the chronic case but there may be some marginal benefit to be obtained from a diet rich in unsaturated fatty acids.

Optic neuritis

Optic neuritis is a common first manifestation of multiple sclerosis and probably nearly every case of multiple sclerosis can expect ultimately to have some evidence of optic nerve involvement. However, every patient who presents for the first time with optic neuritis must be carefully examined to exclude other important causes of damage to the optic nerve such as compression by tumour or aneurysm, drug toxicity, vitamin B_{12} deficiency, neurosyphilis or hereditary optic atrophy.

The immediate prognosis of optic neuritis is favourable, the majority of patients recovering vision completely or nearly completely in the course of a few weeks. The long-term prognosis is less certain as figures in the literature estimating the risk of the patient ultimately developing multiple sclerosis vary from less than 20 per cent to more than 80 per cent. Compston *et al.* (1978) have identified three factors which significantly increase the probability that a patient with optic neuritis will develop multiple sclerosis in the future. The first of these is positive typing for HLA antigen BT101 which occurs in a high proportion of patients with multiple sclerosis. This antigen is closely related to, and may be identical with, HLA-DRw2. The second factor is onset of the attack in winter in patients showing positive typing for BT101, and the third is the factor of recurrent attacks. On this basis the risk of developing optic neuritis as the first manifestation of multiple sclerosis would seem to be greatest in a genetically susceptible individual exposed to an infective agent prevalent in the winter months. Previous studies by McAlpine (1964) and Bradley and Whitty (1968) suggest that multiple sclerosis which follows an initial episode of optic neuritis tends to manifest a clinically mild course.

A number of studies have indicated that treatment with corticotrophin or prednisolone leads to a more rapid recovery from the acute attack of optic neuritis but suggest that eventual recovery of vision is no more complete in treated than in untreated cases (Rawson *et al.*, 1966; Bowden *et al.*, 1974; Gould *et al.*, 1977). Treatment with steroids therefore remains a matter for individual judgement but there is clearly a strong indication when visual loss is bilateral or pain about the eye is a prominent feature.

Treatment of complications

1. *Care of the bladder*

The commonest disturbance of bladder function in multiple sclerosis is urgency of micturition. This is associated with hyperactivity of the micturition reflex and the bladder tends to be of small volume. On the other hand in other patients the bladder reflexes are affected and this may lead to hesitancy of micturition; eventually the bladder becomes atonic and distends passively to give rise to overflow incontinence. Sometimes patients with multiple sclerosis develop acute retention of urine and this is not infrequently the presenting feature in an acute exacerbation. In all these conditions infection may aggravate the symptoms and in the atonic bladder urinary stasis may lead to stone formation which forms an additional focus for infection.

Whatever the cause of bladder dysfunction it is important to maintain an adequate fluid intake and to treat episodes of infection with the appropriate antibiotic. If there is urgency of micturition it may be helpful to advise the patient to empty the bladder every two hours by the clock and further relief may be obtained by using anticholinergic drugs such as propantheline bromide (probanthine) 15 mg three times a day, or emepronium bromide (cetiprin) 100—200 mg three times a day. If there is hesitancy of micturition the patient may learn to assist bladder emptying by pressure over the abdomen and help may be given by cholinergic drugs such as bethanechol chloride (myotonine) 10 mg three times a day or distigmine bromide (ubretid) 5 mg three times a day. Acute retention may necessitate catheterisation which can be carried out intermittently at first or, if the retention persists, an indwelling catheter can be used. Frequently if retention develops during an exacerbation of multiple sclerosis it will eventually subside spontaneously. If retention develops as the first feature of an exacerbation urological investigation is advisable to exclude some local pathology in the urogenital system. If hesitancy or retention is persistent it is sometimes possible to relieve it by surgical resection of the bladder neck. Incontinence in the male patient can be managed by the patient wearing a portable urinal which is strapped to the thigh and connected to the penis by a length of condom tubing. This is not possible in the female who may require an indwelling catheter. Sometimes these patients will manage when the incontinence is not severe by wearing plastic pants containing absorbent pads. Once a patient has an indwelling catheter recurrent infection is inevitable and every effort should be made to delay the use of this by careful training and control of infection. In certain patients the most satisfactory situation can be attained by exteriorisation of the ureters through an ileal loop, the urine draining into an external container. This, however, is a fairly major surgical procedure not to be undertaken lightly. Self-catheterisation can be learned by some patients using a 'clean' but non-sterile technique. An 8F or 10F disposable catheter may be used and discarded at the end of the day, or a 12F metal catheter may be employed for long-term use. This technique requires adequate vision and hand control. Urinary infection remains a problem but antibiotics should not be used routinely unless the infection gives rise to symptoms (Lapides *et al.* 1972; *Lancet*, 1979).

2. *Care of the bowels*

Faecal incontinence is a less frequent problem than bladder dysfunction in patients with multiple sclerosis, but if it occurs — as it may in severely disabled patients — it may be relieved by careful training of the patient to defaecate at a fixed time with the aid of a suppository. It is more common for patients to become constipated but it may be possible to control this by the addition of sufficient residue to the diet or, failing this, by the use of laxatives such as senna which can be administered on alternate days. A few patients do not manage with this treatment and require digital evacuation.

3. *Spasticity*

Hypertonicity, particularly of the lower limbs, is a frequent problem in multiple sclerosis. It may take the form of generalised stiffness giving rise to a spastic gait but more frequently the patient will complain of spasms of the muscles, generally of the flexors but sometimes of the extensors. As the condition progresses the limbs may come to occupy a position of continued flexion or extension which can only be overcome with difficulty by passive movement. If spasticity is inevitable it is preferable that the lower limbs should be spastic in extension because then there is some possibility that they will be able to weight-bear, whereas spasticity in flexion may lead to the patient being chairbound or bedridden in a permanently uncomfortable position which makes nursing difficult and increases the risk of pressure sores. Sometimes the posture which the spastic limb develops can be determined to some extent by careful positioning; physiotherapy, in which the patient is taught to walk between parallel bars, may assist in attaining the extended posture as also may lying prone in bed, if the patient can be encouraged to do so. Drug treatment may be helpful but in the ambulant patient if the limbs are in extension excessive treatment with drugs may lead to the limbs becoming flaccid and no longer able to bear weight. The drugs which are helpful include diazepam 6—40 mg per day in divided doses, but high dosage readily gives rise to drowsiness. Dantrolene sodium (Dantrium), which appears to have a relaxant action on the muscle fibres, is made up in 25 mg capsules and the dosage may be increased progressively from 25 mg on the first day up to a maximum of 100 mg four times a day. The patient should be controlled on the smallest dose compatible with relief of spasticity and a limitation with this drug is that muscular weakness may become evident as spasticity is relieved. A particularly useful drug is baclofen (Lioresal). This is related to γ-aminobutyric acid and appears to be particularly effective in spasticity of spinal origin. It is made up in 10 mg tablets, and 15—60 mg daily in divided doses may be given. If severe spasticity in flexion develops it is sometimes possible to relieve this, if other measures fail, by giving an intrathecal injection at the appropriate radicular level of 2—10 per cent phenol in glycerine, or Myodil in doses of 0.5—2.0 ml. If this is done in carefully selected cases spasticity may be reduced with preservation of muscle power. Great care must be taken if bladder function is to be preserved, but the treatment is more generally applicable to patients who have already lost control of bladder function.

4. *Pressure sores*

Normally if a patient maintains a position for any length of time local pressure on any part of the body gives rise to discomfort and the patient automatically moves to take the pressure off the affected part. Where there is sensory loss particularly affecting pain sensation this does not occur and pressure necrosis will readily develop. If sensation is intact the danger is much less, but the pressure points are always at risk if there is severe paralysis or spasticity which prevents corrective movements. In this situation regular changes of position are necessary and the patient must be turned at least as frequently as once every 2 h if he is in bed, and if he is sitting on a chair must be lifted regularly for a few seconds every 15 min. It is essential to inspect all pressure points daily and if there is any sign of redness or bruising the part must be protected from pressure. If a pressure sore has developed the most important measure of treatment is to protect the affected area from all pressure and the strict discipline of turning the patient 2-hourly is essential. Areas of sloughing or necrosis may be removed with eusol dressings. Deep pressure sores may require plastic surgery and skin grafting.

Although there is no substitute for the regular examination and care of pressure areas a number of special beds are now available which contribute to the prevention of pressure sores without imposing a heavy load on nursing staff. These include the large-cell ripple bed, water-beds, sand-beds and the low-air-loss bed (Scales, 1976). These are costly, require skill in operating, and careful maintenance; a relatively simple low-cost bed which can be used in the patient's home is the Egerton net suspension bed (Gibbs, 1977) in which the patient lies in a mesh hammock suspended from rollers so that the patient can be turned easily and rapidly by a single attendant. The Simpson—Edinburgh low-pressure air-bed is another relatively simple bed in which the patient can lie without the same need for frequent turning (McLemont *et al.*, 1978).

In the treatment of established sores a particular problem may be the removal of slough which must be carried out effectively if healing is to take place. If this does not separate easily with eusol or hydrogen peroxide or 0.5% cetrimide, Debrisan, which is composed of microscopic beads of a high molecular weight dextran may be effective although it is expensive (McClement *et al.*, 1979) and lytic enzymes such as trypsin may also be used. Corticosteroids may delay the healing of pressure sores although the injection of a single dose of corticotrophin 80 i.u. has been found to lessen the postoperative incidence of pressure sores in patients undergoing femoral surgery (Barton and Barton, 1976). Incontinence of urine greatly increases the risk of pressure sores and the use of an indwelling catheter may be indicated. Useful adjuvants to therapy are a high-protein diet, ascorbic acid and zinc sulphate, and blood transfusion in patients with anaemia or evidence of protein loss.

5. *Physiotherapy*

If the patient loses the ability to walk during an acute exacerbation careful retraining with the physiotherapist will frequently be successful in mobilising the patient, who progresses from active exercises in bed to walking between parallel bars, then with a Zimmer walking aid, and finally learning to walk independently. Passive movement of the limbs is valuable in relieving spasticity, as is regular exercise of the lower limbs on a stationary bicycle. The ataxic patient may be assisted by walking exercises in improving the gait, and severe ataxia of the limbs can sometimes be helped by having lead weights attached to the distal part (Hewer *et al.*, 1972). Swimming is an excellent exercise which enables the limbs to be used in a non-weight-bearing situation. It is important not to exhaust the patient by over-strenuous sessions of physiotherapy; sometimes the physiotherapy is best administered in courses of 4—6 weeks rather than for extended periods.

6. *Trigeminal neuralgia*

This may occur in multiple sclerosis and is similar in character to the idiopathic form but may occur at a younger age. It frequently responds to treatment with carbamezapine or phenytoin. Sometimes in multiple sclerosis the problem arises that relatively small doses of these drugs will cause ataxia; in this situation the possibility of surgical treatment needs to be considered.

7. *Seizures*

Epileptic seizures are commoner in patients with multiple sclerosis than in the general population but chronic recurrent seizures are uncommon. Occasionally patients have tonic seizures which consist of episodes of unilateral painful muscular spasm sometimes induced by movement; paroxysmal episodes of ataxia or sensory disturbance may also occur. These symptoms frequently respond to treatment with carbamezapine.

General management

The initial episode of multiple sclerosis, particularly if it is one of optic neuritis, is frequently followed by a prolonged remission. At this stage great caution must be exercised in discussing the diagnosis with the patient and certainly this should not be disclosed until it is certain. On the other hand, once the condition is established, it is generally unwise to withhold this information, particularly if the patient has important decisions to consider, such as marriage or having a family.

Pregnancy, trauma, support of social services

Although relapses may be more frequent in the puerperium, careful follow-up of patients who have had pregnancies has shown little adverse effect on the natural history of the disease over an extended period (Millar, 1961; Schapira *et al.*, 1966). In general, however, it is advisable that the patient should become pregnant (if at all) only during a remission. Multiple sclerosis is not in itself a contraindication to the contraceptive pill, nor is it necessarily an indication for termination of pregnancy. Trauma and infection are possible aggravating factors in multiple sclerosis but it is important that in any intercurrent illness the patient should not be confined to bed longer than necessary. Many patients will require the support of the social services. This includes advice on allowances, on the supply of wheelchairs and gadgets for the severely disabled such as the possum apparatus. Alterations can be made to a person's home — such as provision of bath-rails, stair-rails and ramps for a wheelchair — and a careful assessment of the home situation by an occupational therapist will frequently enable suitable measures to be undertaken.

Spinal cord stimulation

In 1973 Cook and Weinstein reported on a patient who had been treated by spinal cord stimulation for the relief of intractable pain. This patient suffered from multiple sclerosis and the treatment was followed by a marked improvement in motor function. Since that time the technique has been studied both in patients with multiple sclerosis and in patients with other neurological disorders, particularly spinal cord injury. Illis *et al.* (1980) have reported on the effects of this treatment in multiple sclerosis, their patients achieving a variable improvement in motor control and a moderate to marked improvement in bladder function. The technique involves implantation of epidural electrodes, and long-term assessment of the patients and further evaluation will be necessary before its place in management can be established.

ACUTE DISSEMINATED ENCEPHALOMYELITIS
(*see also* Chapter 10)

This condition, which may follow an acute virus infection, differs from multiple sclerosis in that it is an acute illness which may have a fatal outcome, complete recovery, or partial recovery with some continued disability, but it does not have a relapsing course. In patients who have continued disability many of the problems which persist are similar to those in multiple sclerosis, and require to be treated along the same lines. In the acute stage there is frequently a favourable response to corticotrophin administered in a programme similar to that recommended for an acute relapse of multiple sclerosis (Miller and Gibbons, 1953).

REFERENCES

Barton, A A and Barton, M (1976) Drug based prevention of pressure sores. *Lancet*, 2, 443–444.

Bates, D, Faucet, P R W, Shaw, D A and Weightman, D (1978) Polyunsaturated fatty acids in treatment of acute remitting multiple sclerosis. *Lancet*, 2, 1390–1391.

Behan, P O, Melville, I D, Durward, W F, McGeorge, A P and Behan, W H M (1976) Transfer factor in multiple sclerosis. *Lancet*, 1, 988–990.

Bowden, A N, Bowden, P M A, Friedmann, A I, Perkin, G D and Rose, F C (1974) A trial of corticotrophin gelatine injection in acute optic neuritis. *Journal of Neurology, Neurosurgery and Psychiatry*, 37, 869–873.

Bradley, W G and Whitty, C W M (1968) Acute optic neuritis: prognosis for development of multiple sclerosis. *Journal of Neurology, Neurosurgery and Psychiatry*, 31, 10–18.

Brody, J A, Sever, J L, Edgar, A and McNew, J (1972) Measles antibody titres of multiple sclerosis patients and their siblings. *Neurology (Minneapolis)*, 22, 492–499.

Carp, R I, Licursi, P C, Merz, P A and Merz, G S (1972) Decreased percentage of polymorphonuclear neutrophils in mouse peripheral blood after inoculation with material from multiple sclerosis patients. *Journal of Experimental Medicine*, 136, 618–629.

Compston, D A S, Batchelor, J R, Earl, C J and MacDonald, W I (1978) Factors influencing the risk of multiple sclerosis developing in patients with optic neuritis. *Brain*, 101, 495–511.

Cook, A W and Weinstein, S P (1973) Chronic dorsal column stimulation in multiple sclerosis. Preliminary report. New York State. *Journal of Medicine*, 73, 2826.

Edie, M J and Tyrer, J H (1980) *Neurological Clinical Pharmacology*. MTP Press Ltd, Lancaster, England.

Field, E J (1966) Transmission experiments with multiple sclerosis: an interim report. *British Medical Journal*, 2, 564–565.

Field, E J and Joyce, G (1979) Multiple sclerosis: what can and cannot be done. *British Medical Journal*, 2, 1571–1572.

Fog, T, Jersild, C, Dupont, B, Platz, P S, Svejgaard, A, Thomsen, M, Midholm, S, Raun, N E and Grob, P (1975) Transfer factor treatment in multiple sclerosis. *Neurology (Minneapolis)*, **25**, 489—490.

Gibbs, J R (1977) Net suspension beds for managing threatened and established bed sores. *Lancet*, **1**, 174—175.

Gould, E S, Bird, A C, Leaver, P K and McDonald, W I (1977) Treatment of optic neuritis by retrobulbar injection of triamicinolone. *British Medical Journal*, **1**, 1495—1497.

Hallpike, J F (1980) New treatments for multiple sclerosis. *Hospital Medicine*, **23**, 63—68.

Hewer, R L, Cooper, R and Morgan, M H (1972) An investigation into the value of treating intention tremor by weighting the affected limb. *Brain*, **95**, 579—590.

Illis, L S, Sedgwick, E M and Tallis, R C (1980) Spinal cord stimulation in multiple sclerosis: clinical results. *Journal of Neurology, Neurosurgery and Psychiatry*, **43**, 1—14.

Lance, E M, Kremer, M, Abbosh, J, Jones, V E, Knight, S and Medawar, P B (1975) Intensive immunosuppression in patients with disseminated sclerosis. *Clinical and Experimental Immunology*, **21**, 1—12.

Lancet (1979) Clean intermittent catheterisation (Leading article), **2**, 448—449.

Lapides, J, Diokno, A C, Silber, S J and Lowe, B S (1972) Clean intermittent self-catheterisation in the treatment of urinary tract disease. *Journal of Urology*, **107**, 458—461.

Lassmann, H and Wisniewski, H M (1979) Chronic relapsing experimental allergic encephalomyelitis. Clinicopathological comparison with multiple sclerosis. *Archives of Neurology*, **36**, 490—497.

Liversedge, L A (1975) Role of steroids and immunosuppressives. In: *Multiple Sclerosis Research*, pp. 261—263. (Eds) A N Davison, J H Humphrey, L A Liversedge, W I McDonald and S S Porterfield. London, Her Majesty's Stationery Office. Amsterdam—New York. Elsevier Publishing Company.

McAlpine, D (1964) The benign form of multiple sclerosis: results of a long-term study. *British Medical Journal*, **2**, 1029—1032.

McLemont, E J W, Shand, I G and Ramsay, B (1979) Pressure sores: a new method of treatment. *British Journal of Clinical Practice*, **33**, 21—25.

McLemont, Elizabeth, Simpson, D C, McCubbin, K J, Dick, T D, Buchan, A C and Harris, P (1979) Simpson—Edinburgh low-pressure air bed: an early clinical evaluation. *Paraplegia*, **16**, 154—159.

Mertin, J and Caspary, E A (1975) Inhibition of the lymphocyte response in multiple sclerosis by linoleic acid. In: *Multiple Sclerosis Research*, pp. 198—207. (Eds) A N Davison, J H Humphrey, L A Liversedge, W I MacDonald and J S Porterfield. HMSO, London.

Millar, J H D (1961) The influence of pregnancy on disseminated sclerosis. *Proceedings of the Royal Society of Medicine*, **54**, 4—7.

Millar, J H D, Vas, C J, Noronha, M J, Liversedge, L A and Rawson, M D (1967) Long-term treatment of multiple sclerosis with corticotrophin. *Lancet*, **2**, 429—431.

Millar, J H D, Zilka, K J, Langman, M J H, Payling Wright, H, Smith, A D, Belin, J and Thompson, R H S (1973) Double-blind trial of linoleate supplementation of the diet in multiple sclerosis. *British Medical Journal,* 1, 765–768.

Miller, H G and Gibbons, J L (1953) Acute disseminated encephalomyelitis and acute multiple sclerosis; results of treatment with ACTH. *British Medical Journal,* 2, 1345–1348.

Miller, H, Newell, D J and Ridley, A (1961) Multiple sclerosis. Treatment of acute exacerbations with corticotrophin (ACTH). *Lancet,* 2, 1120–1122.

Rawson, M D, Liversedge, L A and Goldfarb, G (1966) Treatment of acute retro-bulbar neuritis with corticotrophin. *Lancet,* 2, 1044–1046.

Rose, A S, Kuzma, J W, Kutzke, J F, Namerow, N S, Sibley, W A and Tourtellotte, W W (1970) Co-operative study in the evaluation of therapy in multiple sclerosis: ACTH versus placebo. *Neurology (Minneapolis),* 20 (2), 1–59.

Rosen, J A (1979) Prolonged azathioprine treatment of non-remitting multiple sclerosis. *Journal of Neurology, Neurosurgery and Psychiatry,* 42, 338–344.

Scales, J T (1976) Air support for the prevention of bed sores. In: *Bed Sore Mechanics,* pp. 259–267. (Eds) R M Kenedi and J M Cowden. Macmillan Press, London.

Schapira, K, Poskanzer, D C, Newell, D J and Miller, H (1966) Marriage, pregnancy and multiple sclerosis. *Brain,* 89, 419–428.

Shatin, R (1964) Multiple sclerosis and geography. New interpretation of epidemiological observations. *Neurology (Minneapolis),* 14, 338–344.

Swinburn, W R and Liversedge, L A (1973) Long-term treatment of multiple sclerosis with azathioprine. *Journal of Neurology, Neurosurgery and Psychiatry,* 36, 124–126.

Thompson, R H S (1975) Unsaturated fatty acids in multiple sclerosis. In: *Multiple Sclerosis Research,* pp. 184–191. (Eds) A N Davison, J H Humphrey, L A Liversedge, W I MacDonald and J S Porterfield. HMSO, London.

Tourtellotte, W U (1975) What is multiple sclerosis? Laboratory criteria for diagnosis. In: *Multiple Sclerosis Research,* pp. 9–26. (Eds) A N Davison, J H Humphrey, L A Liversedge, W I MacDonald and J S Porterfield. HMSO, London.

Zabriskie, J B, Vtermohlen, V, Espinoza, C, Plank, R and Collins, R C (1975) Immunologic studies with transfer factor in multiple sclerosis patients. *Neurology (Minneapolis),* 25, 490.

CHAPTER EIGHT

Tumours and Hydrocephalus

TUMOURS OF THE CENTRAL NERVOUS SYSTEM

Only some benign intracranial and spinal tumours can be treated effectively by surgery. The majority of tumours, predominantly gliomas and metastatic lesions, cannot be excised, and surgery is palliative. In this chapter the techniques of treatment are outlined and then the particular problems presented by each type of tumour are discussed.

Treatments available

1. *Surgical*

The results of surgery of early benign tumours such as acoustic neuroma, meningioma, or pituitary adenoma are excellent. These results are achieved because of improvement in surgical techniques, including microsurgical methods, better radiography, including angiography, CT scanning, and good anaesthesia, which permits prolonged operations with satisfactory cerebral circulation. When confronted by more advanced but benign tumours the surgeon may be forced to accept incomplete removal where a more radical approach is judged to be hazardous. Gliomas can seldom be excised, but occasionally a frontal or anterior temporal tumour may be partially excised as a palliative measure by the removal of tumour bulk to provide short-term internal decompression. If a tumour so distorts the CSF pathways that hydrocephalus develops, a shunt may be used, usually ventriculo-atrial or ventriculo-peritoneal. The insertion of a shunt may be the sole procedure if the tumour is inoperable. Sometimes a shunt is inserted to permit improvement in the patient's condition before a direct approach to an operable tumour.

2. *Radiotherapy*

In radiotherapy high-energy photons produce damage to replicating cells. This may affect both the target tumour and the vascular endothelium. Although radiotherapy has been used intensively for many years its value in some tumours is uncertain. Many studies have been retrospective and poorly controlled. These have reported various treatment regimes with different doses, duration, and extent of treatment. Views have diverged on whether the tumour and immediate surrounding tissue only should be irradiated, whether a more extensive local irradiation is required, or whether the entire neuraxis should be treated. Most studies have followed surgery of varied extent. Success has often been estimated by the length but not the quality of survival. A widely used dosage range is 4500—6000 rad, for above this dose the risk of adverse effects increases considerably. The development of CT scanning may allow more accurate planning of the volume to be irradiated but it is unclear whether this will improve the results. Despite all these difficulties some general conclusions can be drawn from the evidence.

Tumours of a glial origin have moderate to poor radiosensitivity. Malignant gliomas (glioblastoma multiformi) may have a short-term improvement with the 1-year survival better than controls, but this difference largely disappears by 2 years (Deeley, 1974). Astrocytomas are more benign tumours. Radiotherapy increases the 5-year survival from 19 to 46 per cent (Sheline, 1977). Oligodendrogliomas usually have an improved long-term survival. Only 31 per cent survive 5 years without radiotherapy compared to a 5-year survival of 85 per cent with radiotherapy. Both medulloblastomas and ependymomas may spread via CSF pathways and are therefore best treated with irradiation of the entire central nervous system. Pituitary tumours have been treated by radioactive implants or by external irradiation but as surgical techniques have improved its role has become more limited (*see* subsequent section). The radiotherapy of metastatic tumours is unsatisfactory.

The adverse effects of radiotherapy may be immediate or delayed. The early deterioration after high doses arises from vascular damage, oedema and infarction, thereby increasing the mass effect of the tumour. In the rare occurrence of delayed effects a progressive, irreversible, degenerative lesion gradually evolves months or years after the initial treatment. The mechanism of this complication is obscure. When a patient develops further focal signs after irradiation the clinical problem is in differentiating this delayed post-irradiation disorder from a local recurrence of the tumour.

3. Chemotherapy

Although there have been several trials of different therapeutic regimes in glial tumours, e.g. the nitrosoureas, the results have been disappointing and cannot be recommended as standard practice. Combination therapies are now being explored in trials.

4. Treatment of increased intracranial pressure

(a) Assessment. Increased intracranial pressure is defined arbitrarily as pressures exceeding 200 mmH$_2$O (15 mmHg) measured in the lateral decubitus position. High intracranial pressure does not, in itself, produce major problems. Patients may have striking elevation of intracranial pressure in the range of 400–600 mmH$_2$O in benign intracranial hypertension without immediate major neurological signs. The greatest risk with chronically elevated intracranial pressure is that optic atrophy and blindness may occur. Severe clinical problems develop, however, if there is a shift of intracranial structures resulting in ischaemia or compression of vital regions. Clinical observations are vital in the assessment and management of patients with increased intracranial pressure. Brainstem dysfunction presents with vomiting, pyrexia, bradycardia, hypotension or hypertension, respiratory depression, and long tract signs. Pulmonary oedema and ECG changes may occur occasionally. Herniation of the medial temporal lobe at the tentorium may result in IIIrd cranial nerve palsy, hemiparesis, occipital ischaemia from posterior cerebral artery compression, and coma. The abducens nerve is particularly vulnerable to compression. Where there is displacement of intracranial structure slight increases in intracranial pressure may critically worsen the patient's condition. This is most clearly observed during intracranial pressure monitoring when a plateau wave of increased pressure occurs, usually for 5–20 min, during which time the patient's condition may deteriorate. Other less marked oscillations in pressure may also be associated with deterioration, such as the increase which may occur during REM sleep.

Treatment should obviously aim at removing the offending haematoma, benign tumour or abscess, if possible. Cerebral oedema should be treated with osmotic therapy or steroids as discussed subsequently. A shunt may sometimes be required.

(b) Mechanism of brain oedema. Cerebral oedema has been classified into vasogenic, cytotoxic, or interstitial oedema. In vasogenic oedema there is increased capillary permeability, particularly in the white matter, with the extracellular fluid volume increased by a plasma filtrate. The vasogenic oedema that may occur with some cerebral tumours can be more extensive than the tumour itself. Vasogenic oedema may

also occur with cerebral abscess, purulent meningitis, cerebral trauma and contusion, lead encephalopathy and as a component of cerebral oedema after a cerebral infarct.

In cytotoxic oedema the gross metabolic derangement of cells results in intracellular oedema. The extracellular space may be reduced and resistance to perfusion of the microcirculation increases. This cytotoxic oedema may arise from acute hypo-osmolality (dilutional hyponatraemia or inappropriate ADH secretion), cerebral ischaemia or metabolic poisons. Seizures, confusion and coma may occur.

In interstitial oedema there is impairment of CSF reabsorption. Fluid accumulates in extracellular spaces, particularly in periventricular white matter. As neuronal function is little altered there are few clinical manifestations until the disorder is advanced. Benign intracranial hypertension appears to produce interstitial oedema but the mechanisms are obscure.

These types of oedema may co-exist. After cerebral infarction the initial cytotoxic oedema is followed by vasogenic oedema resulting from damage to endothelial cells. In purulent meningitis, cytotoxic oedema may occur accompanied by interstitial and vasogenic oedema.

(c) Osmotherapy. Hypertonic fluids may be used to reduce intracranial pressure rapidly in a critical situation, to allow improvement before an operation. They shrink normal brain but not the area affected by vasogenic oedema. The effects of one or two infusions are short-lived, lasting for hours only, as the solute is rapidly distributed in the body and excreted. An infusion of 25 per cent mannitol in adults over 20 min may produce marked improvement. If there is no improvement with one unit a second is unlikely to help and it is not advisable to give more than two units. A brisk diuresis may occur with marked electrolyte loss. In the ill, electrolyte-depleted patient, this further electrolyte loss may be critical. Urea has been superseded by mannitol. Oral or prolonged parenteral chemotherapy is not useful because the solute enters the region of vasogenic oedema causing a rebound increase in intracranial pressure. Another limiting factor is that the brain adapts to hyperosmolality by metabolic changes which increase the intracellular osmoles, thereby reducing the effective osmotic gradient.

(d) Steroid therapy. Steroids reduce vasogenic oedema by a poorly defined 'membrane-stabilising' effect. It is doubtful that they reduce the tumour size although there is experimental support for this effect when given in massive doses. The effects of dexamethasone 10 mg i.v. or i.m. start in 8–30 h, and are maximal after 3–4 days of continued

therapy with a high-dosage oral or parenteral regime, such as 4 mg t.i.d. or q.i.d. Some patients with gliomas may have improvement which is maintained for months but the dosage should be tapered to the smallest dose that will maintain the patient. A dose of 10 mg dexamethasone is approximately equivalent to 130 mg of prednisolone. Dexamethasone is preferred to other steroids because the mineralocorticoid effects are less than with the alternatives. Nevertheless fluid retention and potassium depletion may occur. Diabetes may be precipitated or exacerbated, gastric ulceration and haemorrhage may occur. Steroid psychosis is relatively uncommon.

5. *General measures*

Seizures should be treated with anticonvulsant drugs (*see* Chapter 2). The terminal illness of a patient with a cerebral tumour is often more distressing for the relatives than the patient who may become confused, euphoric or disinhibited. As it is difficult to deal with a querulous, irritable, moody, or forgetful patient, it may help caring relatives to explain that these behavioural changes are a direct result of the tumour, and not of their awkward handling of a difficult situation. This may relieve guilt and help them with the process of coping with the terminal illness. Whether the patient should be managed at home with the help of a family physician, or in a hospital or hospice, depends on the patients, the family, and the local medical facilities.

Agitation may have to be controlled with a tranquilliser such as chlorpromazine. Cyclizine, metoclopramide, or prochlorperazine may relieve vomiting.

Individual tumours

Glioma

A tissue diagnosis from a biopsy taken at craniotomy, or a needle biopsy, usually establishes the diagnosis. Occasionally when the clinical features, the CT scan, and a tumour circulation on an angiogram are in keeping with the diagnosis, a biopsy is omitted. Small tumours situated in the frontal poles or low in the temporal lobe may be resectable. Most tumours are not surgically treatable but radiotherapy may improve the prognosis as discussed previously. The results are better with low-grade astrocytomas and oligodendrogliomas. Dexamethasone reduces cerebral oedema and a low oral dose may maintain this improvement.

Brainstem gliomas are not surgically treatable, and sometimes a biopsy is not safe. Radiotherapy is the treatment of choice.

Optic nerve gliomas may be excised if small, or treated by radiotherapy if extensive.

A medulloblastoma differs from other tumours in this group in its characteristic position in the midline of the cerebellum extending into the brainstem, and its tendency to spread by forming seedlings throughout the subarachnoid space. Surgical exploration is needed to confirm the diagnosis but is hazardous if the tumour is invading the brainstem. The treatment of choice is radiotherapy. The 5-year survival has been reported as 30–65 per cent.

Cerebellar astrocytoma develops in a slightly older age-group, usually after the age of 10 years. Surgical excision offers the best prognosis, and sometimes a cure.

If an ependymoma presents with hydrocephalus, a shunt is needed. The tumour should then be resected, if possible, and then irradiated.

Meningioma

These benign, slowly growing tumours are sometimes surgically resectable, depending on the size and site. The neurosurgeon may be faced with considerable technical problems in the excision of large, inaccessible or vascular tumours. In some patients a partial removal only is possible, despite the risk of recurrence. In the elderly patient with a small inaccessible tumour it may be wise to refrain from operation. Convexity meningiomas are more easily excised than at other sites. Spinal meningiomas are satisfactorily treated if diagnosed before irreversible cord compression occurs. There are occasional malignant variants with a poor prognosis.

Acoustic neuroma

The results of surgical excision of small tumours *via* a trans-labyrinthine approach are excellent. In contrast, less satisfactory results of surgery are obtained when the tumour has expanded into the posterior fossa producing distortion of the brainstem, cranial nerves and the blood supply. Excision may be at the cost of cranial nerves, particularly the facial and trigeminal nerves, but the brainstem is also at risk. Some surgical centres develop considerable expertise in the treatment of these challenging tumours, and report low morbidity and mortality. In the younger patient with a large tumour a total excision may be attempted, whereas in the older patient the less radical intracapsular excision may be acceptable as recurrence is less likely during the life of the patient.

Miscellaneous other tumours

Cerebellar haemangioblastomas

These are uncommon tumours that present with ataxia, nausea, vomiting and headache. As brainstem signs are more likely to arise from compression than direct infiltration by the tumour they must not be interpreted as indicating an untreatable problem. Excision should include the tumour nodule in the wall of the cyst to prevent recurrence. Radiotherapy is indicated in the occasional patient with massive, highly vascular, irremovable tumours. These tumours may co-exist with polycythaemia, or tumours at other sites — in the spinal cord, lung, kidney or liver (Lindau disease).

Microgliomatosis (primary CNS lymphoma)

This condition may be confirmed with a biopsy, but the tumour is too widespread for excision. Radiotherapy is the treatment of choice and the tumours are more radiosensitive than other primary cerebral tumours.

Choroid plexus papillomas

These develop in any of the ventricles and present with hydrocephalus either from obstruction of CSF pathways or, rarely, from excessive production of CSF. They require a shunt and/or excision.

Colloid cysts of the 3rd ventricle

These are uncommon tumours which present with symptoms of increased intracranial pressure and hydrocephalus and/or disturbances of hypothalamic function. Headache, confusion or coma may develop rapidly if hydrocephalus develops acutely; if the position of the colloid cyst changes to allow resolution of the hydrocephalus, improvement may occur, at least for a time.

CT scanning is very useful in the diagnosis of both choroid plexus papillomas and colloid cysts of the 3rd ventricle. Direct excision is difficult, but should be attempted. Shunt procedures may be hazardous as the tumour expands.

Dermoid and epidermoid cysts

These are rare tumours developing in a variety of intracranial sites, in subarachnoid cisterns, particularly the parapontine and chiasmal, and within the lateral or 4th ventricle. Some are excised easily while others that present with hydrocephalus may require to be shunted also.

Pineal tumours

Pineal tumours are rare and vary considerably in their histological features. Pineoblastomas are highly malignant tumours of undifferentiated histology which may develop in childhood, and sometimes disseminate widely throughout the CSF pathways. Radiotherapy is the treatment of choice, and irradiation of the entire neuraxis is recommended because of the spread. Pineocytomas may develop at any age, and differentiate to varying degrees towards astrocytes, ganglion cells, or both. Some relatively undifferentiated pineocytomas may be malignant, although less so than the pineoblastomas. The differentiated tumours occurring in later life are more benign and remain localised. Surgical excision is fraught with danger, and radiotherapy is the treatment of choice. If there has been compression of the aqueduct resulting in hydrocephalus a shunt procedure is indicated.

Chordomas

Chordomas arise in the sacrococcygeal region or the basisphenoid expanding into the sphenoid, basi-occipital bone, the paranasal sinuses, the sella turcica, and cavernous sinuses. The presenting problems vary considerably as the tumours may present with visual symptoms, posterior fossa signs, raised intracranial pressure or nasopharyngeal obstruction. Treatment is unsatisfactory. Chordomas are seldom excisable and they are relatively radioresistant.

Glomus jugulare tumours

These may present with aural symptoms only, or they may encroach on any of the cranial nerves between the 5th and 12th. A small tumour presenting in the middle ear is totally resectable. Surgery in the more extensive lesions is difficult for these highly vascular tumours are sometimes impossible to resect totally. The place of radiotherapy is difficult to assess as it has been used most commonly in addition to surgery. Success has been reported with radiotherapy only (Thomson *et al.*, 1975) and if the low relapse rate after irradiation is confirmed radiotherapy will be more satisfactory than extensive and possibly incomplete resection.

Pituitary tumours

Pituitary tumours must be carefully assessed for both endocrine function and extension to involve the optic chiasm. Accurate visual field recording is important to establish if there has been expansion out of the pituitary fossa. Plain X-rays, tomography of the pituitary fossa, CT scanning and sometimes, in addition, angiography or air encephalography may outline the extent of the tumour. The merits of surgery or radiotherapy for chromophobe, acidophil, or basophil adenomas are controversial. The transphenoidal excision of microadenomas within the pituitary fossa is effective, has a low mortality and morbidity and is the treatment of choice in most centres. The alternative is to use proton-beam therapy which also has a low risk of recurrence, but this technique is restricted to few centres. If there is suprasellar extension the surgical approach is by a transfrontal route. If the removal is incomplete or the patient is unfit for surgery then radiotherapy must be used. Surgery is performed under steroid cover. The need for long-term replacement treatment is determined after the operation. Diabetes insipidus may occur post-operatively, is usually transient, and careful maintenance of fluid balance is needed. Follow-up assessment of visual fields, pituitary fossa X-rays and the endocrine state is required to detect recurrence of the tumour.

Bromocriptine, an ergot derivative, is a dopamine agonist which reduces growth hormone and prolactin secretion. There have been a few reports that it may reduce tumour size. As information is not available concerning its long-term use, it cannot be recommended as a treatment of choice for adenomas secreting either growth hormone or prolactin. There may be a place for bromocriptine in treating the rapid tumour expansion which may occur during pregnancy, and for treating patients unfit or unwilling to have surgery. The dosage is 2.5 mg b.d.

Craniopharyngiomas

These tumours occur most commonly in childhood and present with endocrine abnormalities, visual symptoms or increased intracranial pressure. The most satisfactory tumours to treat are the rare intra-pituitary, or small infra-infundibular ones as they may be excised with microsurgical techniques. The commoner large, invasive, and vascular tumours provide major surgical problems. Cysts can be decompressed and hydrocephalus from 3rd ventricular obstruction may require a shunt. Decompression of visual pathways is important. Radical excision of large tumours has had some firm advocates, but the mortality is high and a number of patients have recurrences on follow-up. Surgery may be complicated by stupor, other mental changes or endocrine abnormalities. Steroid cover is usually required and this should be followed by careful assessment of the need for long-term supplementary hormone treatment. There is some evidence that postoperative radiotherapy delays the onset of recurrence. Attempts at local radiotherapy with injection of radioisotopes into the cysts have been reported but the value remains uncertain.

Nasopharyngeal tumours

These are usually carcinomas or sarcomas which infiltrate the base of the skull producing deafness, facial pain, diplopia, dysarthria and headache. They cannot be excised and radiotherapy is palliative.

Cerebral metastases

Cerebral metastases from systemic tumours, usually from the bronchus or breast, are often untreatable. Some patients present with an apparently isolated large metastatic lesion but pathological findings usually show that it is accompanied by smaller intracranial lesions. Occasional successes have been reported in the excision of a single neoplasm but where the primary tumour is untreatable, or there are metastases elsewhere, surgery is not indicated.

Dexamethasone may produce a striking temporary improvement. Another palliative treatment is radiotherapy with 2500—5000 rad to the brain over 3—4 weeks. The 1-year survival is very poor at about 10 per cent. Systemic chemotherapy also produces unsatisfactory control of intracerebral metastases.

Carcinomatous meningitis, diagnosed with CSF cytology, has an appallingly poor prognosis. Treatment is not indicated if there is disseminated malignancy elsewhere, but should the patient's problems arise only from carcinomatous meningitis, intrathecal methotrexate (10—20 mg on alternate days) or cytosine arabinoside (35—50 mg on alternate days) may be used. If there is no improvement after three or four doses further treatment is unlikely to help. Intrathecal chemotherapy may be combined with irradiation of the neuraxis.

The management of leukaemias of the central nervous system with radiotherapy and intrathecal cytotoxic drugs is covered in reports on the management of leukaemias.

HYDROCEPHALUS

CSF is secreted by the choroid plexuses and to an uncertain extent by ependymal linings of the ventricular system at a rate of about 0.35 ml/min, which is maintained remarkably constant despite increases of CSF pressure. The rate of absorption of CSF is dependent upon the pressure gradient between CSF and the intracerebral venous system. Although the term 'hydrocephalus' describes an increase in the volume above the normal 130–140 ml in adults this is not the only criterion for diagnosis. The increased CSF volume that accompanies the cerebral atrophy of Alzheimer's disease, after head injury or a cerebral infarction, are to be differentiated from hydrocephalus in which there is a failure of removal of CSF, accompanied by an increase in pressure. Excessive CSF production by a choroid plexus papilloma is an extreme rarity. High-pressure hydrocephalus causing headache, nausea, vomiting and altered consciousness may complicate a congenital abnormality, a tumour or defective CSF absorption after meningitis, head injury or subarachnoid haemorrhage. The increase in CSF pressure is marked in contrast with the minor or episodic increases in the so-called 'normal-pressure' hydrocephalus.

Drugs which reduce CSF production, e.g. acetazolamide, have limited duration of action and are rarely effective. The treatment is, therefore, surgical, either removing the obstruction such as an intraventricular or posterior fossa tumour, or the insertion of a shunt which diverts the CSF from the ventricles to the right atrium or peritoneum. The Torkildsen procedure which produced a shunt from the ventricular system to the basal cisterns is seldom used now. Occasionally in communicating hydrocephalus a shunt from the spinal subarachnoid space to the peritoneum is feasible. The improvement in headache, vomiting and mental function after shunting may be rapid, within hours or days, or a slower improvement over many weeks or months may occur in 'normal-pressure' hydrocephalus. The best results are obtained in patients in whom the clinical deterioration had been present for only a short time.

Diagnosis

CT scanning is a non-invasive method of showing hydrocephalus clearly and supersedes air encephalography. Hydrocephalus is differentiated from cortical atrophy by the prominent ventricular dilatation and the relative absence of cortical sulci. CT scanning may also show associated cystic lesions such as porencephaly or a Dandy-Walker cyst.

Complications of shunt procedures

(1) Obstruction of a shunt may occur at the ventricular end from infection, debris or the choroid plexus. Blockage may occur at the atrial end from thrombus or in the peritoneum by adhesions.

(2) Thromboembolism may occur from atrial shunts, resulting in pulmonary embolic lesions which are usually asymptomatic although pulmonary hypertension may occur. The superior vena cava may develop partial or complete occlusion.

(3) A low-grade or florid ventriculitis or meningitis may occur. Infection of the catheter tip in the atrium may result in a thrombotic endocarditis. Even vigorous antibiotic therapy is usually unsatisfactory and the infected shunt has to be removed.

(4) Subdural haematomas may occur.

'Normal-pressure' hydrocephalus (low-pressure hydrocephalus)

The diagnosis should be considered in patients with intellectual impairment, a gait disorder, and/or micturition difficulties, particularly if there is a history of trauma, subarachnoid haemorrhage, or meningitis. After Hakim and Adams (1965) described the syndrome many demented patients with incontinence and gait disturbance were shunted. The results of this unselective surgery were disappointing and the diagnostic criteria now need to be considered carefully. Three approaches have been used. Intracranial pressure monitoring may record intermittent increases in pressure. Secondly, defects of CSF absorption may be sought using either the rate of reabsorption of radioisotope-labelled albumin from the CSF or the pressure recordings produced by infusion of standard volumes of artificial CSF. The third approach is an anatomical one, measuring the ventricular dilatation and prominence of the sulci on CT scanning. The most reliable indicator of subsequent improvement has been controversial but is probably intracranial pressure monitoring. The small oscillations in pressure, often lasting for 30—120 s (the saw-tooth or B-waves of Laundau), and more prolonged elevations in pressure indicate a potential for improvement after shunting in patients who have been shown to have hydrocephalus on CT scanning.

Congenital malformations

The major clinical problems produced by developmental anomalies of the brain and spinal cord in neonatal life are not discussed here. Lesser anomalies, particularly of the hindbrain and upper cervical cord, may present in childhood and adult life. Hydrocephalus from aqueduct stenosis, posterior fossa cysts, or failure of development of the foramina between the 4th ventricle and the subarachnoid space are satisfactorily investigated with CT scanning, and require either a shunt or an exploration of the posterior fossa.

Syringomyelia

Ideas about the pathogenesis of syringomyelia have evolved in recent years with the recognition of its association with posterior fossa and upper spinal cord developmental anomalies, the Chiari malformations (for review *see* Barnett *et al.*, 1973). In addition to the sensory dissociation, the upper limb wasting, weakness and autonomic impairment, and the lower limb spasticity, patients may have clinical features arising from the associated hydrocephalus or syringobulbia. Skeletal abnormalities may be present but the cervical spine X-rays are often normal. Myelography with myodil in prone and supine positions, or air myelography, usually confirm the syringomyelia and upper cervical anomaly. These anomalies and also basal arachnoiditis cause progressive cystic dilatation of the cervical cord and the syringomyelia may be improved by surgery in which the foramen magnum is explored and the abnormalities decompressed. The precise procedure depends on the findings at operation and the surgeon's preference. The results are much better than direct attacks on the syrinx itself.

If syringomyelia complicates spinal cord trauma cystotomy may improve patients with partial cord lesions. More radical surgery may be needed for syringomyelia above a complete cord transection. Syringomyelia associated with spinal tumours or spinal arachnoiditis is seldom helped by surgery.

REFERENCES

Barnett, H J M, Foster, J B and Hudson, P (1973) *Syringomyelia*. Saunders, London.

Deeley, T J (1974) Localised treatment to the brain. Modern Radiotherapy and Oncology. In: *Central Nervous System Tumours*. (Ed) T J Deeley. Butterworths, London.

Hakim, S and Adams, R D (1965) The special problems of symptomatic hydrocephalus with normal cerebrospinal fluid pressure. Observation of cerebrospinal fluid hydrodynamics. *Journal of the Neurological Sciences*, 2, 307–327.

Sheline, G E (1977) Radiation therapy of brain tumour. *Cancer*, 39, 873–881.

Thomson, K, Elbrond, O and Anderson, A P (1975) Glomus jugulare tumours. *Journal of Laryngology and Otology*, 89, 1113–1121.

CHAPTER NINE

Infections of the Nervous System

Infections of the nervous system present varied and challenging problems in diagnosis and management. Infections are common where malnutrition and poor social conditions are present. Infections are also more common when immune competence is impaired as with malignant diseases or immunosuppressive therapy, but often treatment of the underlying disorder is unsatisfactory. Immunisation is important in several infections but is not discussed here. Neonatal infections are omitted, and tropical, fungal and parasitic infections discussed only briefly.

BACTERIAL INFECTIONS

Bacterial infections are often more effectively treated than viral, fungal or protozoal infections, but their management demands rapid, precise clinical and bacteriological diagnosis and a prompt start of antibiotic therapy.

Meningitis

Clinical and pathological considerations

The infecting organism should be identified, if possible, urgently. The clinical features may give some guide. A petechial or purpuric rash suggests a meningococcal infection although a similar rash may occasionally occur with pneumococci. Pneumococcal infections are more common where there are focal infections in the lungs, sinuses or a fracture of the base of the skull. In children under the age of 3 *Haemophillus influenzae* meningitis is common. Immune deficiency states may predispose to infection with a variety of organisms some of which are unusual, such as *Listeria monocytogenes*. Associated urinary tract infections may suggest Gram-negative infections.

Examination of CSF obtained at lumbar puncture is the most important investigation. This should give a bacterial diagnosis, antibiotic sensitivities, and measurements of protein, glucose and cells.

The inflammatory changes spread from the meninges to involve the adjacent brain resulting in confusion, coma or seizures. If there is inadequate or late treatment death or persistent neurological deficits such as epilepsy, mental retardation, spasticity, blindness or deafness may occur. Three pathological changes are important in treatment. The first is that the meningeal inflammatory reaction results in increased permeability to some drugs which would otherwise penetrate to the brain poorly, e.g. penicillin, streptomycin. In contrast, isoniazid, sulphonamides and chloramphenicol cross the blood—brain barrier relatively easily. Cerebral oedema is another pathological consequence of meningitis that may complicate treatment. Occasionally blockage of CSF pathways and hydrocephalus occurs as a late effect and a shunt is needed.

The dramatic neurological manifestations should not obscure the recognition of systemic features, particularly in meningococcal and staphylococcal infections. Blood cultures should be done. The systemic complications of septicaemia, hypotension, peripheral circulatory collapse and renal failure must be treated.

General measures

Intensive nursing care is essential. When vomiting or shock is present, intravenous fluids are required and drugs are given parenterally. Fever is treated with tepid sponging. Aspirin or paracetamol are helpful if they can be taken.

Seizures may result directly from the meningitis, from neurotoxicity after massive doses of penicillin, or from electrolyte disturbances, in particular, hyponatraemia. Diazepam may be used for status epilepticus or very frequent seizures (*see* Chapter 2) and correction of hyponatraemia or reduction of penicillin dosage may be indicated. Longer-term treatment with anticonvulsants (phenytoin, carbamazepine or sodium valproate) may be needed. Phenytoin should be started with a loading dose (*see* Chapter 2).

If cerebral oedema causes life-threatening tentorial or cerebellar herniation mannitol 20 per cent i.v. can be used for its rapid action (*see* Chapter 8). Dexamethasone provides the slower onset of a more prolonged response but may impair the host response to the organism and reduce the penetration of some antibiotics. Steroids therefore have limited value in the treatment of meningitis.

Meningococcal meningitis

The variable prognosis probably reflects the patient's inherent immune mechanisms. At its worst the patient may die within hours of the onset, but in the more slowly evolving infections, developing over 2—3 days, the prognosis is better.

Examination of CSF should show Gram-negative cocci both intracellularly and extracellularly, together with a raised cell count and protein concentration and reduced glucose. Blood cultures may also be positive.

The antibiotic of choice is benzyl penicillin G given by i.v. bolus infusions. A reasonable regime in adults is to give 4-hourly infusions of 2 megaunits for 7—10 days. At the first lumbar puncture 5000—20 000 units of penicillin may be given according to the age. Large-volume i.v. infusions may produce problems. Potassium penicillin may produce cardiac arrhythmias if infused too rapidly and the sodium salts of penicillin may exacerbate fluid retention. In very high dosages seizures sometimes occur from a direct toxic effect of penicillin when the dose exceeds 24 megaunits daily, but it is more likely with doses over 48 megaunits daily.

Although sulphonamides were effective drugs in previous decades resistant organisms are now so widespread that these drugs are little used. The dose of sulphadiazine is 3 g i.v. as a loading dose followed by 1.5 g 4-hourly for 48 h then 1 g 4-hourly. Adequate fluid intake and urine output must be maintained and the treatment changed to oral therapy in 24—48 h if the patient is well enough. There is some evidence that even a large single dose may be effective in a population with sensitive organisms.

Cephaloridine 1 g 6-hourly in adults together with intrathecal doses of 50 mg daily for 3 days, or preferably, chloramphenicol 1 g 6-hourly in adults, 100 mg/kg per day in children, are alternative regimes for use in the penicillin-sensitive patient.

As the mechanisms in the catastrophic Waterhouse—Friderichsen syndrome are uncertain it is not surprising that the management is unsatisfactory. Disseminated intravascular coagulation occurs and the value of heparin is uncertain. While heparin may be used early, the risk of haemorrhage increases in advanced cases. Despite the striking adrenocortical lesions these patients do not have low plasma cortisol levels and additional steroids probably do not improve the prognosis, and indeed may worsen it. Fluid and electrolyte balance requires careful attention as the patient may become oliguric. Both dehydration and overhydration are to be avoided.

Prevention.   The close contacts of the patient are vulnerable and chemoprophylaxis should be used as soon after establishing the diagnosis as is feasible. Rifampicin 600 mg b.d. for four doses in adults or 10 mg/kg in children may be given. Minocycline 200 mg, then 100 mg b.d. for 5 days is an alternative but it may produce vertigo. If the organism is known to be sulphonamide-sensitive, sulphadiazine 2—3 g daily can be used. Vaccines are available against some serotypes (A, C) but not for the commonest infection in the UK and the USA which is serotype B.

Pneumococcal meningitis

Penicillin is the antibiotic of choice, given by i.v. bolus injections as for meningococcal meningitis. This is combined with daily intrathecal penicillin for 7 days, with a dose in adults which must not exceed 20 000 units. The most satisfactory alternative drugs are the cephalosporins and they may yet prove to be superior to penicillin. Cephaloridine is at least as good and possibly superior to penicillin (Love *et al.*, 1970). It can be given intrathecally 50 mg in adults, 25 mg in children, 12.5 mg in infants and systemically 100 mg/kg. The total daily dose should not exceed 6 g. Newer cephalosporins may prove to be better, e.g. cephuroxime or cefotaxime. Chloramphenicol or erythromycin are further alternatives.

Recurrent meningitis

This usually occurs where there is an anatomical defect, often in the cribriform plate or middle ear, or when there is an immune deficiency. These patients require careful investigation for occult CSF leak or fistula as this demands surgical closure to reduce the risk of further recurrence.

Haemophilus influenzae meningitis

This infection is commonest in children under the age of 5 years in the UK, but is a commoner cause of meningitis in adults in many countries, including the USA and Australia. The treatment of choice is chloramphenicol starting in adults with 1 g i.v. 6-hourly, and in children 100 mg/kg (neonates should not receive more than 50 mg/kg daily). There have been some cases of chloramphenicol resistance.

Ampicillin in large doses of 75—150 mg/kg daily i.v. is an alternative to chloramphenicol, but in some regions resistance makes this antibiotic an inappropriate choice. The newer cephalosporins such as cephotaxime may be used.

A less common alternative is streptomycin intrathecally and intramuscularly together with sulphonamides.

Staphylococcal meningitis

This infection may complicate ventricular shunts, cranial injuries, spinal abscess, or staphylococcal infection at other sites. As many organisms produce penicillinase, methicillin or flucloxicillin should be used intravenously. Alternatively lincomycin or cephaloridine may be used.

Listeria meningitis

Occasional infections with *Listeria monocytogenes* occur in adults, especially the elderly and the immunosuppressed, either in the form of meningitis or abscess (Lechtenberg *et al.*, 1979). Ampicillin, at least 150 mg/kg daily in divided doses, or chloramphenicol, are the most satisfactory antibiotics but penicillin given intravenously in very high doses, erythromycin or tetracycline are alternatives.

Gram-negative bacterial meningitis

Gentamycin systemically and intrathecally may be given together with chloramphenicol. With *Pseudomonas aeruginosa* sodium carbenicillin may be combined with gentamycin. The intrathecal route for gentamycin is used for the refractory or severely ill patients at a dose of 4—8 mg daily but the ventricular concentration may still be low. If necessary ventricular administration may be given *via* a surgically implanted reservoir. The systemic dose of gentamycin is 1.0—1.5 mg/kg 8-hourly. The serum levels should be monitored, especially if renal function is impaired. Carbenicillin is given in a dose of 0.5 mg/kg daily divided into 4-hourly doses. Cefotaxime has had encouraging initial reports (Belohradsky *et al.*, 1980).

Meningitis where the organism is unknown

Where the patient clearly has a bacterial meningitis, but no organism has been seen on examination or cultured from the CSF, treatment is given to cover the most likely organisms. Penicillin and chloramphenicol or cefotaxime have quite broad ranges of action and are therefore reasonable choices, especially in the child.

If there is a chronic meningitis with no evidence of tuberculosis on Ziehl—Neelsen staining, negative VDRL and stain for cryptococcus, a therapeutic trial of antituberculous therapy should be considered. If there is no improvement, a trial of antifungal treatment should be given.

Tuberculous meningitis

As tuberculosis has declined in developed countries tuberculous meningitis has become a rarity except perhaps in Asian immigrant communities. The subject has been well reviewed by Parsons (1979). The clinical features usually evolve gradually. These include headache, nausea, vomiting, cranial nerve palsies, confusion and coma. General nursing and supportive measures are needed. The contentious areas in management concern the choice and routes of administration of antibiotics and the use of steroid treatment. The fall in numbers of patients in recent years has made it difficult to assess the newer antibiotics. Therefore some doubt remains about their use and the optimum duration of therapy. Treatment for 2 years now appears unnecessary and a 12—18-month course is adequate.

The drugs of choice are now isoniazid, rifampicin and streptomycin in combination. The drugs should be started before drug sensitivities are available and are changed later, if necessary, according to the laboratory results.

Isoniazid passes readily into the cerebrospinal fluid. It may cause a sensory neuropathy from altered pyridoxine metabolism in patients who acetylate the drug slowly and should therefore be accompanied by pyridoxine 10 mg daily. It should be given to adults in a dose of 400—500 mg daily. Children may start with the higher dose of 10—15 mg/kg daily for 8 weeks, reducing then to 5 mg/kg.

Rifampicin crosses the blood—brain barrier adequately only when inflammation is present. It is likely to become less effective as the patient recovers. The dose is 450—600 mg daily orally in adults and 10—20 mg/kg daily in children. Ethambutol has a limited place and its value has not been clearly established. It crosses to the brain relatively poorly and therefore a high dose of 25 mg/kg daily is needed. This dose is reduced to 15 mg/kg after 2 months because of the risk of retrobulbar neuropathy. Streptomycin is an effective drug but has to be given parenterally (0.75—1 g daily in adults and 200 mg—1 g in children). After 2—3 months the dose is reduced to 1 g two or three times weekly. As it is transported poorly to the brain, an intrathecal route has been widely used. The value of intrathecal injections is, however, controversial. Some studies have reported improvement only when intrathecal streptomycin is introduced. In this regime, 100 mg daily in adults or 25–50 mg in a child for 2 weeks has given the impression of a rapid response in severely ill patients. As the consequences of inadequately treated tuberculous meningitis are so severe it is argued that this route should be used until a more satisfactory regime is firmly established. Opponents of this view simply record that many patients recover satisfactorily without an intrathecal route. There have been no controlled trials. Intrathecal streptomycin may cause a pleocytosis so that the number of cells in the CSF cannot be taken as an indication of the response to treatment. If a cisternal route is being used because of spinal block, the concentration should be halved because of the risk of ototoxicity.

In the patient with organisms resistant to the drugs of choice, ethionamide and cycloserine may be considered. Both readily enter the CSF. With ethionamide 10–15 mg/kg daily, hepatic toxicity and gastrointestinal disturbances are prominent. The psychosis and the liability to seizures limit the use of cycloserine (15 mg/kg daily).

The use of steroids has been controversial. They are clearly indicated for severe cerebral oedema, severe drug reactions, and adrenal failure. Debate has centred on whether they reduce or prevent the development of the basal exudation and fibrosis and the arteritis which results in cranial nerve palsies, hydrocephalus, and cerebral infarction. The clinical evidence for their benefit is, on the whole, poor. Mortality is reduced but the survivors are severely brain damaged. The clearest indication for attempting to reduce fibrotic inflammatory changes is when the patient is developing spinal block. Steroid treatment carries three additional problems. It suppresses the usual clinical and CSF responses to infection making the evaluation of the response to treatment difficult. It may mask other infections, including secondary bacterial meningitis. There is also a risk that reducing the permeability of the blood–brain barrier towards normal may reduce the transport of rifampicin and streptomycin to the brain and the CSF. Steroid therapy carries the usual complications of fluid retention, ulcers, psychosis, etc. which are discussed in standard therapeutic texts.

Purified protein derivate (PPD) given intrathecally was claimed to reduce intracranial inflammation, but has been used little outside the originating neurological centre, possibly because it is complex to use, with important adverse effects.

Assessing the response to treatment. A few days after the start of treatment, the white cells in the CSF, mainly polymorphonuclear leucocytes, increase owing to massive release of tuberculin into the CSF. The CSF protein concentration also increases. As clinical improvement gradually occurs in subsequent weeks, the glucose concentration rises while the cells and the protein in the CSF, the temperature and ESR gradually fall. The protein may remain high for over 6 months. A graph makes the progress easier to assess. Occasionally a shunt may be needed for hydrocephalus (*see* Chapter 8). In spinal tuberculosis, if paraplegia evolves rapidly or occurs despite antibiotic therapy, surgical exploration and decompression should be considered.

BRAIN ABSCESS

The incidence of brain abscess has fallen in recent years making the diagnosis easy to overlook. The mortality and morbidity in published series remains high despite modern diagnostic and surgical techniques and antibiotic therapy.

Diagnosis in relation to treatment

CT scanning has the advantage of providing rapid, accurate localisation without hazard to the patient. Hydrocephalus, oedema (a low-density area) and distortion of cerebral structures can be seen. After contrast enhancement the ring-like area of increased density may be particularly striking. Supratentorial abscesses show better than infratentorial ones. Where CT scanning is not available, isotope scans may be used, followed by angiography.

Lumbar puncture is not to be recommended in the management of these patients for three reasons. Firstly, normal CSF does not exclude an encapsulated abscess. Secondly, the changes of increased protein and cell count are non-specific, contributing neither to the localisation nor to the identification of the offending organism. Thirdly, it is potentially hazardous. In one series a number of patients without overt signs of increased intracranial pressure deteriorated after lumbar puncture (Garfield, 1969). The main indication is for the exclusion of possible purulent meningitis.

For many years bacteriological studies have reported 'sterile' pus in some abscesses, but this is likely to have arisen from poor handling of the pus. A recent study (De Louvois *et al.*, 1977a) reported the isolation of an organism in all cases provided that pus taken at operation is handled appropriately using standard techniques. Inoculation must be done rapidly into both aerobic and anaerobic media.

Treatment

Surgery

The aim of treatment is the urgent evacuation of pus. Some surgeons drain the pus only, while others prefer complete excision of the abscess. This decision depends, in part, on the duration of the abscess. Excision is impossible before the abscess has become clearly localised, with an organised wall. If the abscess is secondary to chronic mastoiditis, radical mastoidectomy should be performed early. If the patient is deteriorating, with signs of herniation, urgent treatment with mannitol may be needed to allow time for investigations and preparation for surgery.

Antibiotic therapy

Abscesses associated with infected sinuses are often caused by *Streptococcus milleri* or *Strept. pneumococci*, both of which are penicillin-sensitive. However, antibiotic penetration into an abscess is poor. Some of the penicillin may be inactivated by the pus. For these reasons high doses of penicillin are needed (16—24 megaunits daily). The duration of treatment is uncertain but should probably be more than 4 weeks.

Post-traumatic and spinal abscesses are usually caused by *Staphylococcus aureus*, which produces penicillinase. As cloxacillin and cephaloridine penetrate poorly into the abscess, fusidic acid has been recommended as the treatment of choice (De Louvois *et al.*, 1977b). The dose is 500 mg of sodium fusidate in 250—500 ml saline infused i.v. over 2—4 h three or four times daily. Spinal abscesses require decompression.

Abscesses secondary to middle ear infections are usually in the temporal lobe or cerebellum, and often contain a mixed growth of organisms. These bacteria include the Bacteroides group, Proteus and various Streptococci. High doses of systemic antibiotics are needed based on antibiotic sensitivities at culture. Sometimes treatment needs to be started empirically with chloramphenicol, penicillin G and methicillin (or cloxacillin). Gentamycin may be needed for the Gram-negative organisms. Metronidazole penetrates reasonably well and has a place in the mixed growth secondary to middle ear infections.

Septic cerebral sinus thrombosis

Thrombosis complicating suppuration may occur in sagittal, cavernous and lateral sinuses. The main treatment is surgical drainage of infected sinuses or abscesses. As the organisms are usually *Staph. aureus*, Streptococci or Pneumococci the antibiotics should include methicillin or cloxacillin in high dosage.

Steroids

There have been no clinical studies but an experimental study (Quartey *et al.*, 1976) showed reduced elimination of the organism when steroids were combined with specific antibiotic therapy. The formation of the fibrous wall around the abscess was also impaired. The implication is clear. Steroids are to be avoided if possible unless definitive clinical studies show their benefit.

Assessment of the response to therapy

Changes in the size of the abscess, the extent of oedema and the distortion of the intracranial structures are most satisfactorily followed by serial CT scans. If CT scanning is not available, the established method is to place a small amount of Myodil in the abscess cavity and follow the changes on plain X-ray during subsequent weeks.

Epilepsy

Unfortunately, the risk of seizures is high both during the acute infection and subsequently. The incidence of epilepsy after abscess has been variously reported as between 30 and 50 per cent. It may be delayed in its onset between 1 month and 15 years (Legg *et al.*, 1973).

SPINAL ABSCESS

Paraplegia or quadriplegia may evolve rapidly and, as with other spinal lesions, urgent investigation with myelography is required. The important treatment is surgical decompression combined with antibiotic therapy.

NEUROSYPHILIS

Although the numbers have declined dramatically neurosyphilis still occurs and may present diagnostic problems. The presentation may be atypical, perhaps because of previous partial inadvertent antibiotic treatment. In addition, physicians are perhaps less aware of the diagnosis than in previous generations. Some male homosexuals are now thought to be especially at risk as the primary and secondary stages of the illness may be missed.

Serological and CSF examinations are needed. The Wasserman test has been largely supplanted by another non-specific test, the VDRL test. The fluorescent Treponema antibody absorbed (FTA—ABS) test and the *Treponema pallidum* haemagglutination test are more specific tests for *Treponema pallidum*.

Drugs

Penicillin is the treatment of choice. A prolonged high-dose course is needed because penetration to the brain is poor. The minimum dose and duration is still uncertain. A widely used regime is to give 1 mega-unit (600 mg) of procaine penicillin G i.m. for 21 days. It is uncertain whether benzathine penicillin is as effective as procaine penicillin G. Unfortunately, despite this high dose, there may be recurrences and therefore review is needed in the early years after treatment. Refractory cases should be admitted to hospital for more intensive treatment with a 10-day course of 12—24 megaunits of benzyl penicillin i.v. (2—4 megaunits every 4 h). If a patient is allergic to penicillin, the alternative regimes are erythromycin 500 mg 6-hourly for 15 days repeated at monthly intervals for 3 months, tetracycline 3 g daily for 3 weeks or cephaloridine 2 g daily for 21 days. As experience with these regimes is limited there is no clear basis for recommending an alternative of choice.

The Herxheimer reaction

This systemic reaction may follow the start of even a small dose of an antibiotic. The mechanism is uncertain and its occurrence unpredictable. It may be more common in general paralysis of the insane (GPI) than in other forms of late syphilis. Fever, flushing, sweating, headache and malaise may last for several hours and rarely in tertiary syphilis there is an exacerbation of the patient's condition, probably due to ischaemia in affected regions. Patients with optic neuritis may be given prednisolone as prophylactic treatment, 5 mg q.i.d. for a day before starting penicillin or hydrocortisone hemisuccinate 200 mg i.v. may be given before the first dose.

Assessing the response to treatment

Variable clinical improvement occurs. In severe paretic and tabetic problems, and in juvenile syphilis, the prognosis is poor. Milder paretic presentations and meningeal forms with high cell counts are more likely to improve. Evidence for a response to treatment should be sought and the patient reviewed periodically for evidence of recurrence. The earliest guides to success are the fall in lymphocyte count in the CSF in 6—12 weeks, followed by a decline in protein concentration in 3—6 months. Positive serological tests may subsequently become negative but in late syphilis they may remain positive despite treatment, and cannot therefore be taken as a criterion of successful therapy. Another persistent abnormality is elevation of CSF globulins (or IgG or the Lange curve). It is reasonable to follow a course of treatment with lumbar punctures at 6 weeks, 6 months and 1 year, repeating the antibiotic treatment if the cell count or protein fail to fall or, having fallen, increase again, or if the serological tests become more abnormal. A persistent pleocytosis is associated with a poor prognosis.

Other problems

The clinical problems are quite diverse. The 'lightning' pains of tabes dorsalis can sometimes be controlled with mild analgesics — for example, aspirin or paracetamol — and powerful addictive analgesics such as opiates are not advisable. Sometimes carbamazepine or phenytoin may help. Steroids have been reported to be occasionally helpful but should not be used long-term.

Tabetic autonomic crises can be difficult to manage. In a gastric crisis abnormalities of fluid and electrolyte balance must be corrected. Adrenalin 0.5 ml 1/1000 s.c. or ephedrine 30—60 mg orally may help. Laryngeal crises may be helped with inhalation of amylnitrate. Painless retention of urine may occur in tabes dorsalis and catheterisation is needed. Charcot's arthropathy should be treated with orthotic devices to relieve stress on the affected joint, if possible. Surgery on these joints produces unsatisfactory results and is seldom indicated. Attention to foot hygiene and the treatment of corns and callosities by chiropody is important to prevent ulceration of the foot. If perforating ulcers do occur, pressure should be taken off them as for other pressure sores.

Syphilitic optic atrophy should be treated with prednisolone 30—60 mg daily, in addition to penicillin, to halt the deterioration in visual acuity. Careful repeated measurements of visual acuity and the visual fields are needed to assess progress.

TETANUS

The neurotoxin of *Clostridium tetani* affects reflex activity in the spinal cord and brainstem, possibly by interfering with the inhibitory action of Renshaw cells. This produces generalised or localised muscle spasm often involving co-contraction of agonists and antagonists. In severe cases, sympathetic over-activity causes tachycardia, labile hypertension and peripheral vasoconstriction. Many cases arise from very minor or even unrecognised wounds, but if a wound is present it should be excised if possible. The patient should receive i.v. penicillin in large doses such as 1 megaunit benzyl penicillin 6-hourly for a week. The value of antitoxins has been unclear from clinical trials but the balance of evidence is in their favour, and therefore immunoglobulin such as human anti-tetanus immunoglobulin should be given (Humotot 30—300 i.u./ kg i.m.).

Further management varies with the severity of the case but management is best in an intensive care unit. Mildly affected cases do not require ventilatory assistance. Sedation with diazepam and chlorpromazine may be sufficient. Noise and movement should be minimised. In more severely affected patients, intensive care is required with intubation followed by tracheostomy if recovery is not prompt. Some patients can then be managed with diazepam, if necessary, in very large doses. If ventilation is impaired or the severe spasms cannot be otherwise controlled curarisation and assisted ventilation is needed. Sympathetic over-activity may complicate the management of the severely affected patient. Although it may be tempting to use β-blockade with propranolol, some patients have developed alarming bradycardia and cardiac arrest during tracheal suction, probably exacerbated by propranolol. Even the severely ill patients may recover satisfactorily and in one large series the 10 per cent mortality rate was from the complications of intensive care rather than directly from the tetanus (Edmondson and Flowers, 1979).

BOTULISM

The neurotoxins of *Clostridium botulinum* produce a rare but dramatic block of neuromuscular transmission resulting in paralysis. As this may emerge within a few hours, urgent treatment is needed. This may include assisted ventilation if the patient can reach suitable facilities soon enough. Antitoxins neutralise the unbound toxins and are therefore used, but do not reverse the binding at the neuromuscular junction. Guanidine may enhance acetylcholine release but its value is doubtful. Antibiotics are not helpful with intestinal infections. If the botulism arises from an infected wound thorough cleansing and debridement is indicated.

MISCELLANEOUS SYSTEMIC INFECTIONS WITH NEUROLOGICAL COMPLICATIONS

Many systemic infections may invade the nervous system. Some, such as malaria, trypanosomiasis and schistosomiasis, are common disorders in tropical countries and therefore very important. Others occur in Western countries but are uncommon, often presenting with a chronic meningitis or meningoencephalitis, e.g. cryptococcus and toxoplasmosis. A full discussion of their management is not appropriate but some points are made about treatment where the nervous system is affected. For more comprehensive discussion of uncommon infections the reader is referred to Murphy *et al.* (1979).

Fungal infections

Infection with *Cryptococcus neoformans* is rare and about half the patients have impaired immunity. It may present as meningitis, encephalitis or an expanding focal lesion. A firm bacteriological diagnosis must be sought with specific request from bacteriological laboratories to use staining with Indian ink preparations, special culture methods or the demonstration of anticryptococcal antibodies in blood and CSF.

The treatment has been unsatisfactory. The most widely used drug is amphotericin B which has to be given parenterally in a prolonged course and carries unpleasant adverse effects. A generally recommended regime is to start with 0.1—0.25 mg/kg dissolved in 5 per cent dextrose in water in a 4 h i.v. infusion followed by further infusions in the subsequent 5 days with gradual daily increments to 1.0—1.5 mg/kg. Thereafter a maintenance regime of thrice-weekly infusions of 0.6 mg/kg can be given until a total 2—3.5 g is given. Some centres measure the peak serum concentration, aiming to give a concentration of 2—2.5 μg/ml. This demanding course may be complicated by a variety of adverse effects: nausea, anorexia, pyrexia with rigors, cardiac arrhythmia, hypotension and weakness. As local thrombophlebitis is likely to occur at infusion sites these should be changed. A little heparin can be added to each infusion (0.5 unit/ml). Antihistamines and hydrocortisone may reduce severe problems. Renal damage is the most serious effect and careful monitoring of renal function is necessary. Reduction in dosage is needed if renal function deteriorates. Amphotericin B may be given intrathecally, starting with 0.025 mg with daily increments to 0.5—1.0 mg well diluted in CSF. Thereafter this dose is given three times weekly. Its value is, however, uncertain and it may be complicated by a chemical meningitis and arachnoiditis.

Two alternatives to amphotericin B are 5-fluorocytosine and micazole. The sensitivity of Cryptococci to 5-fluorocytosine varies and resistant strains rapidly develop when the drug is used alone. This drug should be given orally 150 mg/kg in four divided doses, or smaller doses if renal function is impaired. It may cause nausea, vomiting, diarrhoea, liver and haemopoietic damage. A combination with amphotericin B allows a smaller, shorter course of amphotericin B therapy, and a combined regime is recommended.

Micazole has been successful in sites other than the nervous system but penetrates to the brain relatively poorly. Therefore in addition to either i.v. infusions of 600 mg in adults or an oral dose of 25 mg/kg daily in two divided doses, it has been given intrathecally or intraventricularly (15 mg). The systemic effects may be nausea, vomiting, dizziness, rashes and haematological problems, while the intrathecal route may result in arachnoiditis. A recent series reported success when used intrathecally and intravenously in patients unsuccessfully treated with amphotericin B (Sung *et al.*, 1978).

Candida and Aspergillosis are both opportunist infections which invade the CNS when immunity is impaired. They present with headache, fever, drowsiness, coma, seizures or focal signs. Both are difficult to eradicate but amphotericin B and 5-fluorocytosine may be used, as discussed above.

Toxoplasmosis

This infection by *Toxoplasma gondii* arises most commonly by crossing the placenta. Infections in later life may occur rarely, often in the immunosuppressed patient, causing ocular damage or chronic encephalitis. These may be treated with spiramycin or preferably with pyrimethamine 0.5 mg/kg daily together with a sulphonamide, such as sulphadiazine 30–50 mg/kg daily for 21 days. Haematological control is needed at follow-up on these regimes. Prednisolone may help if vision is critically impaired.

Acute cerebral malaria

This life-threatening manifestation of malaria may present with seizures or with a confusional state, which progresses to coma. Intensive nursing and medical care are needed. Quinine is the treatment of choice in many parts of the world (South America, South-East Asia, parts of Africa) where chloroquine resistance occurs. In addition it is possibly more effective than chloroquine in the patient in coma. Quinine should be given as an i.v. infusion over 4 h at a dose of 10 mg/kg (base) up to 490 mg, repeated in 12—14 h. In small children or those with severe systemic complications smaller doses or less frequent administration is wise.

The alternative is to use chloroquine in an i.v. infusion over 4 h in a dose of 5—10 mg/kg every 12—24 h.

There is uncertainty about the value of steroids. If the patient does not improve with quinine within 24 h, acute cerebral oedema may be present which responds to i.v. hydrocortisone 100 mg 6-hourly or to dexamethasone. Disseminated intravascular coagulation may occur but its management is uncertain. Heparin increases the risk of cerebral haemorrhage and is not to be used. Cerebral perfusion may be impaired and some improvement may occur with a plasma expander, dextran, 500 ml in 24 h. Blood transfusion is to be avoided unless the anaemia is profound. Seizures should be treated with anticonvulsants, initially diazepam. The diazepam may also be useful for the irritability and restlessness which may occur.

After the treatment of the acute illness pyrimethamine and sulpha-doxime (Fansidar) or, alternatively, mefloquine should be given in a single dose.

Trypanosomiasis

A chronic encephalopathy may develop months or years after the initial infection. The treatment is unsatisfactory as most drugs are relatively ineffective or toxic. Melarsoprol (Mel B) is used for the encephalopathy with incremental i.v. doses. Arsenical toxicity may occur. The systemic infection should be treated with suramine, starting with an initial low dose of 0.2 g in case there is an idiosyncratic reaction to the drug. It should then be followed 24 h later by doses of 20 mg/kg i.v. repeated weekly for 4 weeks.

Amoebiasis

The rare cerebral abscesses that complicate intestinal infection with *Entamoeba histolytica* are difficult to treat because drug penetration to the brain is poor. Both emetine and chloroquine, useful in systemic infections, are unsatisfactory. The drug of choice now is metronidazole 800 mg t.i.d. for at least 10 days, but probably up to 6 weeks.

Amoebic meningoencephalitis occurs rarely in two forms. One presents with acute purulent meningitis caused by *Naegleri fowleri* contracted by swimming in warm, stagnant water. It may respond to early energetic treatment with amphotericin B. The other presentation is of a rare chronic granulomatous encephalitis caused by Acanthamoeba. The prognosis is even worse than for the acute disease as there is no established treatment. Metronidazole, sulphonamides, emetine and chloroquine have been used.

Helminth infections

A variety of helminth infections occur in which CNS involvement is only part of a more widespread infection. These include toxocariasis and trichinosis. Thiabendazole may be used for trichinosis in the first 7 days, and later is ineffective. This is unsatisfactory as the infection is usually diagnosed after about 2 weeks, at which stage aspirin and sometimes steroids may reduce the inflammatory reaction in muscle.

Schistosomiasis

The acute or chronic encephalopathy, myelopathy or local lesion may be treated with niridazole, or stibocaptate. Niridazole should be given in a dose of 25 mg/kg orally daily in two divided doses for 10 days. Stibocaptate should be given in a dose of 6–10 mg/kg i.m. weekly. Delay in treatment may result in permanent damage. Steroids may help in acute stages in combination with more specific treatment.

Cysticercosis

Invasion of the brain by the cysticerci from *Taenia solium* may present many years later with epilepsy or with spinal or other focal features. The infection cannot be eradicated and the management is that of the presenting clinical problems — epilepsy with anticonvulsants, hydrocephalus with shunts, and spinal compression with surgical decompression.

VIRAL DISEASES

The great success in recent decades in the prevention of poliomyelitis contrasts with the unsatisfactory results for the treatment of established viral infections of the nervous system. Invasion of the nervous system with viruses may result in meningitis, encephalitis and demyelination. Despite much research, the only viral infections for which chemotherapy is established is in herpes simplex and herpes zoster infections. The use of interferon will be of considerable interest.

Meningitis

Meningitis may be a feature or complication of a variety of viral infections. It generally has a benign course and recovery occurs without residual damage. A small proportion of patients may have visual impairment, convulsions, weakness, sensory symptoms and drowsiness during the acute illness. A few of these patients may have residual weakness.

Encephalitis

Although mild cases occur, viral encephalitis may result in severe brain damage or death. The pathology is either a direct invasion by the neurotropic viruses or an immunologically determined demyelinating process. General nursing and supportive measures are needed with control of seizures and cerebral oedema.

General care

Intensive nursing care with attention to nutrition, hydration, hygiene and care of the skin is essential in the unconscious patient. Four further problems require special mention. Firstly, a difficult problem of judgement may arise in the patient with such severe damage that ventilation is impaired. In herpes encephalitis, the outlook at this stage is grim, and recovery, if at all, is likely to be with severe residual damage. This needs to be borne in mind in the decision as to whether to provide assisted ventilation. Secondly, the control of fluid and electrolyte balance may be complicated by inappropriate ADH secretion, the management of which is discussed in Chapter 10. Thirdly, the risk of seizures is high. If they occur phenytoin, carbamazepine or valproate should be introduced. Status epilepticus should be treated with diazepam or clonazepam (*see* Chapter 2). Fourthly, cerebral oedema can be life-threatening and treatment should be with dexamethasone 10 mg parenterally and 4 mg q.i.d. in subsequent days. There is a theoretical risk that the steroid treatment might impair an immune response to the invading viruses, but the importance of this risk is difficult to evaluate, and may be outweighed by the need to treat severe cerebral oedema.

Herpes simplex encephalitis

The prognosis is poor in this necrotising encephalitis. The mortality is high and the morbidity in survivors is great. The possibility that there may be effective treatment has led to the development of good diagnostic techniques in brain biopsies, using immunofluorescent studies and viral culture. Unfortunately, the less invasive methods of serological or CSF examination do not provide reliable information when a diagnosis is needed, early in the course of the illness. Angiography, the EEG, and CT scanning may all show highly suggestive features but the definitive investigation is brain biopsy. Brain biopsy was advocated before the toxic drug idoxuridine was given systemically, but now with a less toxic drug it is debatable whether a biopsy should precede the start of treatment.

The drug of choice now is adenine arabinoside which, in a controlled trial, reduced the mortality from 70 per cent in a control group to 28 per cent in the treated group (Whitley *et al.*, 1977). The authors thought it unethical to continue the trial once this finding emerged so that the numbers were not sufficient for statistical analysis of the morbidity. The trend appeared to be towards a reduction in the morbidity as well as mortality. Adenine arabinoside was more effective in patients treated early, while drowsy or confused but not unconscious. Therefore if the diagnosis is likely treatment should be started promptly, withdrawing the drug if the diagnosis is not confirmed at brain biopsy. The dose used was 15 mg/kg daily for 10 days given by i.v. infusion over 12 h. Adenine arabinoside is rapidly converted into a deaminated metabolite which can cross the blood—brain barrier. It has a short half-life of 3.3 h and as it is largely excreted in the urine a lower dose may be required in patients with renal failure. Mild reversible granulopenia or thrombocytopenia, anorexia, nausea, vomiting or diarrhoea may occur. There are no major adverse effects. A similar drug, cytosine arabinoside, has given disappointing results.

A much more benign neurological complication of herpes simplex infection is a transient sacral radiculopathy and proctitis in homosexual males (Samarasinghe *et al.*, 1979). Pain, paraesthesiae and rectal discharge disappear within 21 days. The only measure which may be needed, apart from analgesics, is catheterisation if urinary retention occurs.

Herpes zoster infections (shingles)

Vesicles and severe pain are the main problems in herpes zoster infections. If these occur in the ophthalmic division of the trigeminal nerve, threatening vision, topical application of idoxuridine should be used and secondary bacterial infection should be treated with antibiotics. Some claims for the benefits of amantadine in shingles have been made but the evidence for its benefit is scanty. Analgesics are required for the acute phase but the most important complication is the intractable pain of post-herpetic neuralgia (*see* Chapter 6). There are, however, other rare complications of shingles. Sacral herpes zoster, although self-limiting, may cause urinary retention for which catheterisation is needed. Occasional motor deficits such as facial palsy usually recover satisfactorily spontaneously. Meningoencephalitis may complicate trigeminal herpes infection. Severe cases should be treated with cytosine arabinoside 3 mg/kg by i.v. infusion in the first day followed by 2 mg/kg daily for another 3 days (Juel-Jensen, 1973). This regime has not been subjected to rigorous trial.

Post-infectious demyelinating disorders

An acute encephalopathy, myelopathy, radiculopathy or neuropathy may follow viral infections such as measles, mumps, varicella, rubella or immunisation for smallpox or rabies. This is an immunologically determined group of disorders in which the pathology is acute demyelination and mononuclear cell inflammatory reaction. Severely affected patients with encephalomyelitis should be treated with steroids. Acute nursing care, bladder care or physiotherapy are needed (*see* Chapter 7).

Poliomyelitis

Fortunately the widespread use of vaccines has made poliomyelitis rare in Western communities. In a polio epidemic, patients with mild non-specific illness should be nursed quietly, avoiding undue muscular activity. Intensive nursing care is needed for the acute paralytic illness. Aspirin or other mild analgesics can be used. Sedatives should be avoided in borderline ventilatory failure. If respiratory failure occurs, assisted ventilation is needed. Physiotherapy, initially with passive joint movements only should be followed by a programme of active rehabilitation. Orthopaedic procedures become important later when the extent of residual weakness has become clear.

Rabies

The dramatic manifestations and inevitable death of the patient with established rabies are understandably frightening. Public health measures in the control of the spread of infection are important. The immediate management of the patient exposed to a risk of rabies depends on the type of contact and the certainty of exposure. All wounds should be rigorously cleansed and anti-tetanus serum should, if available, be infiltrated in the wound if this is deep. Primary suturing should be delayed. If the animal is suspected as rabid, immunisation is started immediately. It can subsequently be stopped if rabies is not confirmed in the animal. If rabies is confirmed in the animal the course of immunisation is completed and anti-rabies serum is given. If the animal cannot be observed or is a confirmed case, then anti-rabies serum is given from the start with the beginning of vaccination. Vaccines are now prepared from viruses cultured in duck embryo or from various tissue cultures, such as human diploid cells. The vaccination is by s.c. injection and the duration depends on the type of vaccine. The advantage of the newer vaccines is that the risk of neurological complications with neuropathy, radiculopathy or encephalomyelopathy are less than with the earlier vaccines prepared from neural tissue. The duck embryo vaccine is given in 14–21 daily injections. The human diploid cell antigen produces good antibody responses and few adverse effects. It is given as 1 ml s.c. for six doses on days 0, 3, 7, 14, 30 and 90.

The treatment of the established cases is aimed at relieving distress.

REFERENCES

Belohradsky, B H, Bruch, K, Geiss, D, Kafetzis, D, Marget, W and Peters, G (1980) Intravenous cefotaxime in children with bacterial meningitis. *Lancet*, 1, 61–63.

De Louvois, J, Gortvai, P and Hurley, R (1977) Bacteriology of abscesses of the central nervous system: a multicentre prospective study. *British Medical Journal*, 2, 981–984.

De Louvois, J, Gortvai, P and Hurley, R (1977) Antibiotic treatment of abscesses of the central nervous system. *British Medical Journal*, 2, 985–987.

Edmondson, R S and Flowers, M W (1979) Intensive care in tetanus: management, complications and mortality in 100 cases. *British Medical Journal*, 1, 1401–1404.

Garfield, J G (1969) Management of supratentorial abscess: a review of 200 cases. *British Medical Journal*, 2, 7–11.

Juel-Jensen, B E (1973) Herpes simplex and zoster. *British Medical Journal*, 1, 406–410.

Lechtenberg, R, Sierra, M F, Pringle, G F, Shucart, W A and Butt, K M H (1979) *Listeria monocytogenes*: brain abscess or meningoencephalitis. *Neurology*, 29, 86–90.

Legg, N J, Gupta, P C and Scott, D F (1973) Epilepsy following cerebral abscess – a clinical and EEG study in 70 patients. *Brain*, 96, 259–268.

Love, W C, McKenzie, P, Lawson, J H, Pinkerton, I W, Jamieson, W M, Stevenson, J, Roberts, W and Christie, A B (1970) Treatment of pneumococcal meningitis with cephaloridine. *Postgraduate Medical Journal*, 46, (Suppl.), 155–158.

Murphy, F K, Mackowiak, P and Luby, J (1979) Management of infections affecting the nervous system. In: *The Treatment of Neurological Disorders*. (Ed) R W

Rosenberg. S.P. Medica and Scientific Books, New York and London.

Parsons, M (1979) *Tuberculous Meningitis*. Oxford University Press, New York and London.

Quartey, G R C, Johnston, J A and Rozdilsky, B (1976) Decadron in the treatment of cerebral abscess. An experimental study. *Journal of Neurosurgery*, 45, 301—310.

Samarasinghe, P L, Oates, J K and MacLennan, I P B (1979) Herpetic proctitis and sacral radiculopathy — a hazard for homosexual males. *British Medical Journal*, 2, 365—366.

Sung, J P, Campbell, G D and Grendahl, J G (1978) Miconazole therapy for fungal meningitis. *Archives of Neurology*, 35, 443—447.

Whitley, R J, Soong, S-J, Dolin, R, Galasso, G J, Chi'en, L T and Alford, C A and the Collaborative Study Group (1977) Adenine arabinoside therapy of biopsy-proved herpes simplex encephalitis. *New England Journal of Medicine*, 297, 289—294.

CHAPTER TEN

Metabolic, Toxic and Inflammatory Disorders

A variety of inflammatory, metabolic and endocrine disorders some-times affect the nervous system but their management is discussed here only when neurological complications occur. Chronic intoxication from a variety of sources, particularly heavy metals, is discussed, but the management of acute drug overdosage is not.

METABOLIC DISORDERS

Diabetes mellitus

There is now evidence that good control of diabetes in the insulin-dependent diabetic is associated with fewer complications. The primary aim is the accurate control of blood glucose, but research is now also focused upon the control of other metabolic derangements. Diabetes mellitus may be complicated by neuropathy (Chapter 12), stroke (Chapter 3) and coma. The general management of coma is discussed in Chapter 1.

1. Ketotic diabetic coma

Monitoring of electrolyte concentration, glucose and pH is required. A precipitating disorder such as an infection, if present, should be treated. Dehydration should be corrected using i.v. saline, often 1—3 l. Dextrose 5 per cent can be used when the blood glucose falls to 10—11 mmol/l. The electrolyte deficit should be corrected with the addition of potassium chloride to the infusion fluid, monitoring the serum potassium. Sodium and chloride is replaced with saline infusions. Soluble insulin is given either in small frequent doses, e.g. 10 units i.v. and 10 units i.m. repeated hourly (5—10 units) while monitoring the descent of the blood glucose or in larger doses of insulin 4-hourly.

2. *Hypoglycaemic coma*

Hypoglycaemic coma must be rapidly reversed with 10—40 g of 50 per cent glucose given i.v. If a vein cannot be found 1 mg of glucagon may be given i.m. Prolonged severe hypoglycaemia may cause cerebral oedema. Sometimes i.v. mannitol improves this oedema rapidly while dexamethasone results in a more gradual improvement. The benefits of both of these measures are limited because the main form of oedema is cytotoxic with intracellular oedema, and not vasogenic oedema (*see* Chapter 8).

Non-ketotic coma

In this disorder of the elderly the coma may be preceded by seizures, drowsiness, confusion, and apparent stroke. The main aim is to correct the marked increase in osmolality of the blood that arises from grossly elevated glucose concentrations and sometimes from hypernatraemia. Hypotonic saline is infused and the decrease in blood glucose, sodium, and osmolality is monitored. The insulin requirement is usually low, often in the range of 30—100 units only. The blood glucose should be lowered gradually to around 10 mmol/l. Precipitating drugs should be withdrawn, and infection or cardiac failure treated.

Hepatic encephalopathy

Hepatic failure produces a complex, poorly understood metabolic disorder in which a number of possible biochemical changes and impaired cerebral blood flow contribute to the severe neuronal dysfunction. The mainstay of treatment is still the reduction of dietary protein, and the correction of fluid and electrolyte abnormalities. Initially, protein is removed from the diet, and reintroduced gradually when there is improvement to a maintenance level of 40—50 g daily. Adequate calorie intake in the form of carbohydrate, preferably 1500—2000 cal, should be given in the form of i.v. dextrose or *via* a nasogastric tube. Nitrogenous products of bacterial activity in the gut are reduced by treatment with neomycin 1 g q.i.d. As opportunist infections, e.g. Candida, may supervene during prolonged use, neomycin is better reserved for use in the acute encephalopathy rather than in a chronic disorder. An alternative treatment is the use of lactulose which acidifies the gastrointestinal contents, reduces ammonia absorption and is a laxative. It is given orally or *via* a nasogastric tube as a 50 per cent solution of 10—20 ml t.i.d. It should be used in patients who are intolerant of, or refractory to, neomycin. Some patients find it unpalatable for chronic use.

Fluid depletion, hyponatraemia, and potassium depletion need correction. Diuretics should be avoided if possible. Barbiturates, opiates, and other CNS depressants are contraindicated. Associated infection, a possible precipitant of the encephalopathy, must be treated.

Other therapies are still of uncertain value. L-dopa may have an arousing effect. Alpha-ketoglutarate may be used but its value is unclear. A promising recent report is that bromocriptine, up to 15 mg daily, produced neurological improvement and increased cerebral blood flow in a small group of patients with chronic hepatic encephalopathy (Morgan *et al.*, 1980).

Renal failure

Many neurological problems may complicate renal failure.

Uraemic encephalopathy

The clinical features are diverse and the treatment is the control of the uraemia.

Seizures

When seizures arise from the uraemic encephalopathy itself, the treatment is dialysis. Epileptic attacks may also arise as part of the disequilibrium syndrome in acute haemodialysis and they are prevented by decreasing the rate and increasing the frequency of dialysis. Some centres give phenytoin routinely in acute dialysis. Seizures may, however, be secondary to hyponatraemia, hypomagnesaemia, or hypocalcaemia, and these electrolyte disturbances need to be treated. If fits complicate hypertensive encephalopathy, the blood pressure should be reduced urgently but not excessively. Anticonvulsants are required in patients if correction of the metabolic abnormalities is impossible or ineffective. As phenytoin is metabolised in the liver, the dosage is usually normal or only slightly reduced. As the plasma-binding is reduced in renal failure, the proportion of free phenytoin increases and the patient is more likely to become intoxicated as the serum levels increase. Laboratories usually estimate the total phenytoin level but the result is nevertheless useful in assessing dosage. As phenobarbitone is eliminated in the kidneys the dosage needed is less and serum levels provide a useful guide to the requirements. The plasma-binding of sodium valproate is reduced but it is unclear whether this is of practical importance in the management of seizures. Carbamazepine, being less protein-bound and metabolised in the liver, is given in the usual dosage range. Diazepam (or clonazepam) is the treatment of choice for patients with status epilepticus.

Neurological problems with haemodialysis

(a) Dialysis dementia

There is now good evidence associating this condition with high levels of aluminium in the brain. As it is an irreversible, progressive disorder prevention is most important. Aluminium levels in the water used for making dialysate should be very low. In areas with high aluminium content in domestic water deionisers may be used to reduce the aluminium concentration. Whether renal transplantation prevents the progressive deterioration is uncertain. There are isolated reports of improvement after a transplantation.

Diazepam has been reported to improve the speech disorder, an early and prominent feature. The stuttering, non-fluent dysarthria, with some features akin to Parkinsonism, may improve with i.v. diazepam, but some observers have not found a clear response. Diazepam or clonazepam should be used for status epilepticus. Clonazepam or valproate may be used for the long-term control of generalised seizures and clonazepam may reduce myoclonus.

(b) Headache

A throbbing vascular headache, dialysis headache, or an increase in migraine may occur in relation to dialysis and is best prevented by changing the dialysis regime, particularly with more frequent shorter periods of dialysis.

(c) Muscle cramps

Sometimes painful severe cramps may occur during or after dialysis, usually when the dialysate contains a low concentration of sodium. They are best prevented by using higher sodium concentrations, but may be treated with quinine sulphate 300 mg orally, if necessary.

The syndrome of inappropriate ADH secretion

Inappropriate ADH secretion, resulting in hyponatraemia and hypo-osmolality, may complicate a number of neurological disorders —

meningitis, encephalitis, head injury, tumours around the hypothalamic region, acute intermittent porphyria and the Guillain—Barré syndrome. In addition, non-neurological causes such as an oat-cell carcinoma of the lung may present with this metabolic encephalopathy. The clinical features are seizures, agitation, confusion and drowsiness progressing to coma. These abnormalities are much more prominent if hyponatraemia evolves rapidly. In a very slowly evolving syndrome cramp, lethargy, nausea, and anorexia may occur. The biochemical features are a profound hyponatraemia and hypo-osmolality, with high urine osmolality in the presence of normal renal and adrenal function. In these slowly evolving cases, the clinical abnormalities occur when the serum sodium concentration is below 120 mmol/l.

Mild or moderate cases may be treated by encouraging water loss while retaining electrolytes. The fluid intake is restricted severely to around 600 ml daily until the serum sodium returns to normal. Then more fluid may be permitted, up to 1000 ml daily. Supplementary dietary sodium may help but may also precipitate cardiac failure. Democycline 300 mg q.i.d. partially blocks the renal effects of ADH and permits a greater fluid intake (Forest *et al.*, 1978). At this dose it is often nephrotoxic and a t.i.d. dose may be used. Lithium carbonate 250 mg t.i.d. has similar effects.

Severe hyponatraemia and hypo-osmolality can be corrected within hours, if renal function is good, by losing water with a diuretic and replacing the sodium, potassium and chloride lost in the urine (Hartman *et al.*, 1973). It is important to have frequent biochemical analyses of blood and urine. Frusemide 1 mg/kg i.v. is given and hourly collections of urine are analysed for sodium, potassium and chloride. The solute loss is replaced by infusion of hypertonic saline with supplementary potassium chloride over 4—8 h. The desired water loss is calculated thus:

$$\text{desired water loss (litres)} = \text{total body water (weight in kg} \times 0.6)$$

$$- \text{total body water} \times \frac{\text{measured osmolality (nOsmol/l)}}{\text{expected osmolality (270 Osmol/l)}}$$

Another approach for rapid correction of hyponatraemia is to give hypertonic saline infusion. This is an emergency method only, to rapidly correct the hyponatraemia. It may precipitate cardiac failure and as the kidneys excrete the solute load it is of short-term value only.

Acute intermittent porphyria

In this rare condition it is important to avoid precipitating acute attacks by any of the large number of drugs which are contraindicated. These are: alcohol; barbiturates; phenytoin; methsuximide; sulphonamides and griseofulvin; a variety of centrally acting sedative or psychotropic drugs — chlordiazepoxide (Librium), glutethimide, imipramine, meprobamate, dichloralphenazone (Welldorm); ergot preparations; methyldopa. Oral contraceptives are also contraindicated except in a small group of women who have cyclical attacks related to the menstrual period, for in some of these patients oral contraceptives may be helpful. Safe drugs include opiates, corticosteroids, penicillins, streptomycin, tetracyclines, furadantin, phenothiazines, reserpine, guanethidine, diphenhydramine, promethazine, atropine, digoxin, pyridostigmine and neostigmine.

There are no specific measures available for the treatment of an acute attack. A high carbohydrate diet is desirable, as it avoids the exacerbation that occurs in starvation, and this diet may reduce the hepatic δ-aminolaevulinic acid activity. Abdominal pain is treated with chlorpromazine. If the pain persists, opiates may be used provided respiratory depression is not present. Ventilatory failure should be treated with assisted ventilation in an intensive care unit. The hyponatraemia of inappropriate ADH secretion should be treated as discussed in the previous section. Supplementary magnesium may be given if there is hypomagnesaemia. Phenothiazines are used for the psychosis. Seizures may be difficult to control because barbiturates and phenytoin are precluded. Information about carbamazepine and sodium valproate is not available. In the acute attack intravenous diazepam may be sufficient. Clonazepam may be used subsequently although drowsiness often limits its use. As the autonomic nervous system is affected labile hypertension may occur but this seldom requires treatment. Persistent hypertension can be treated with propranolol, guanethidine or reserpine.

INTOXICATIONS

Alcohol

Social and cultural factors are important in causing the major problem of alcoholism but discussion of this important topic is outside the scope of this text. Clearly the long-term solution is abstinence or minimal drinking. This is achieved by the firm resolve of the patient, but he or she usually requires the support of the family and the physician. Admission to an alcoholism unit, or contact with Alcoholics Anonymous or other organisations, may help. Many neurological problems arise from alcoholism.

1. Acute intoxication

A common problem is the assessment of the unconscious intoxicated patient. The effects of alcohol must be differentiated from those of drugs which may have been taken with the alcohol, from head injury, hypoglycaemia, and, in the chronic alcoholic, from Wernicke's encephalopathy. If there is doubt about whether Wernicke's encephalopathy is present, thiamine should be given on its own or, preferably, in a high-potency multiple-vitamin preparation such as parenterovite. Acute intoxication is usually self-limiting, and only rarely results in severe respiratory depression for which intubation and assisted ventilation is required. Forced diuresis is not indicated. Alcohol can be removed by dialysis in critical situations.

2. Alcohol withdrawal

The mild stages of agitation, tremulousness, tachycardia and sweating can be treated with a benzodiazepine such as chlordiazepoxide (Librium) or diazepam. Intercurrent infection must be treated. In a severe withdrawal state there is marked agitation, hallucinations, vomiting, hypothermia, and circulatory collapse. Various regimes have been used to tranquillise these patients. Diazepam or chlordiazepoxide are usually effective. In the acute case diazepam may be administered in 2.5—5.0 mg boluses, repeated if necessary. The usual important hazards are the precipitation of respiratory depression or circulatory collapse. Other successful sedative regimes used are chlormethiazole or chlorpromazine.

3. Withdrawal seizures

These most frequently occur 10—30 h after a prolonged bout of drinking as a single seizure, a run of grand mal seizures or occasionally status epilepticus (Victor, 1970). The EEG is usually normal after recovery from attacks induced only by bout drinking ('rum fits'). If the patient can remain off alcohol, anticonvulsant therapy is unnecessary. A different problem is that alcohol withdrawal, often from modest drinking, may precipitate seizures in patients with epilepsy and in these patients the avoidance of such drinking, and the use of anticonvulsants, is indicated. In addition, the alcoholic is liable to head injury, which may cause epilepsy. Therefore when a seizure occurs after drinking, the history of previous seizures or head injury indicates the need for anticonvulsant drugs.

The use of anticonvulsant drug therapy during voluntary alcohol withdrawal is debatable. If there is a history of previous drug withdrawal fits, phenytoin should be given using a loading dose. A reasonable regime is to give phenytoin 1 g orally over a few hours, then 300 mg daily for 3 days, with a subsequent gradual reduction in dose in the next week.

4. *Wernicke's encephalopathy*

This disorder occurs most commonly in alcoholics but also occurs rarely as a complication of pyloric stenosis, hyperemesis gravidarum or severe malnutrition. As it is often unrecognised in acute admissions (Harper, 1979) there is a need for an awareness in assessing patients who may be alcoholic. The diagnosis should be considered in any alcoholic, particularly if malnourished, who presents with confusion and memory difficulties, with or without the additional features of ocular palsy, ataxia and neuropathy. The syndrome evolves gradually in some patients with the insidious development of subtle impairment of intellectual function. The most incapacitating defect is the amnestic—confabulatory state — Korsakoff's psychosis.

Diagnostic tests for thiamine deficiency are not generally available and the treatment should be started with parenterovite or thiamine 50 mg i.m. daily without biochemical confirmation of the diagnosis. As a glucose load in a thiamine-deficient patient may precipitate or exacerbate the encephalopathy it should not be given to replace fluids without giving thiamine first. Maintenance therapy is with 10—15 mg thiamine daily.

The diagnosis of Wernicke's encephalopathy may be overlooked in a patient presenting with hypothermia as there are lesions affecting the hypothalamic thermoregulatory centres.

5. *Alcoholic dementia, cerebellar degeneration and neuropathy*

Although the occurrence of alcoholic dementia has been recognised for over a century it has been difficult to separate it from other causes of mental impairment in alcoholics, Wernicke's encephalopathy, hepatic encephalopathy and head injuries. It is, however, a distinct entity and it may even be an early presentation in alcoholism (Lee *et al.*, 1979). There is also evidence that if abstinence is complete partial improvement in intellectual function may occur over many months. Psychometric tests are the most reliable measures in the assessment of alcoholic dementia and there is relatively poor correlation of severity with appearances on CT scanning.

Cerebellar degeneration often arises concurrently with the dementia and the most important measure is abstinence.

When assessing an alcoholic with a peripheral neuropathy both liver disease and nutritional deficiencies have to be considered in each patient. Thiamine and other vitamin deficiencies must be treated. Improvement may occur over several months, and it may be incomplete.

Lead poisoning

Chronic lead poisoning in adults results in a predominantly motor neuropathy with early involvement of the extensor groups, particularly at the wrists. Sensory symptoms may occasionally occur. The encephalopathy which occurs in children, and rarely in adults, requires urgent treatment, especially after acute poisoning. A topical, controversial and still unresolved debate is whether impairment of intelligence and behaviour may occur in children exposed to high environmental lead levels. Obviously the source of lead poisoning must be removed. A mild neuropathy may be treated with oral penicillamine at a dose of 250—750 mg daily. Follow-up should include full blood count estimations for evidence of a blood dyscrasia, and urinary proteins for evidence of a nephrotic syndrome as complications of penicillamine.

Patients with severe neuropathy or with encephalopathy need urgent treatment with parenteral chelating agents. British anti-lewisite (BAL) (dimercaprol) and sodium calcium editate should be used. The toxic metallic ion binds in a more stable manner to the —SH groups of BAL than to the affected enzymes. BAL is given by deep, sometimes painful, i.m. injection in a 5 per cent solution at a dose of 5 mg/kg for children under the age of 10, or 3 mg/kg for older children and adults. The injections are repeated 4-hourly for the first day, 6-hourly on the second day, 8-hourly on the third, and then continue 12-hourly for a week. Nausea, vomiting, salivation, lacrimation, muscle aches, paraesthesiae, pain, urticaria, tachycardia, and hypertension may occur. Antihistamine drugs may reduce these changes. Sodium calcium editate is given by bolus i.v. infusions of 12.5 mg/kg every 4 h for 5 days. Less frequent infusions lasting 1 h every 12 h have also been used. Hypotension, lacrimation, sneezing, nasal stuffiness, and muscle pains may occur, but the most important serious effect is renal damage; therefore the blood urea should be measured regularly during treatment.

Hyponatraemia from inappropriate ADH secretion may occur. Its management is outlined in a previous section but is complicated because of the requirement for a moderately large fluid intake. Increased intracranial pressure may occur, and if it is life-threatening mannitol may be used. The place of steroids is uncertain.

Chelation rapidly removes about one-half of the lead from soft tissue stores, but not the lead bound in the bones. After the first course of treatment, the bound lead may be mobilised, the serum level rises again and further treatment is required; therefore serum levels should be monitored after the initial therapy. Penicillamine, which is much less toxic and unpleasant, may be preferable for subsequent treatments.

Mercury poisoning

Chronic inorganic mercury poisoning can be treated with BAL as described previously but larger doses, up to 6 mg/kg daily, may be necessary. As N-acetyl-D,L-penicillamine chelates mercury effectively it may be used in the future but the drug is not generally available.

The organic mercury compounds, methyl and ethyl mercury, are waste products in various industrial processes and they are also used as agricultural fungicides. Poisoning results in a severe and largely irreversible neurological disorder. An enterohepatic circulation occurs which permits treatment with cholestyramine to render the mercury unabsorbable in the small intestine. Cholestyramine is given in a daily dose in adults of 16—24 g in divided doses.

In acute mercury poisoning the unabsorbed mercury in the gastro-intestinal tract can be removed by gastric lavage, but special care should be given to the airway. Intubation is required to prevent aspiration if the patient is drowsy or unconscious. Sodium formaldehyde sulphoxylate can be introduced to the duodenum in a 5 per cent solution up to 250 ml with the aim of reducing the mercury salts to a less soluble form. BAL is then administered as for lead poisoning.

Arsenic and antimony poisoning

As with mercury poisoning the aim is to reduce absorption and promote excretion of the poison. Gastric lavage or emesis should be used with care in acute poisoning together with BAL to chelate the metal. A fluid and electrolyte balance must be established and maintained.

Thallium poisoning

Absorption may be decreased by gastric lavage, then the administration of potassium ferric hexacyanoferrate (Prussian blue) 250 mg/kg into the duodenum in divided doses over 24 h.

Organophosphate poisoning

As organophosphates may be absorbed through the skin the clothing should be removed and the contaminated skin washed. Recent ingestion should be treated with gastric lavage, but only after intubation in any patient with impairment of laryngeal reflexes or drowsiness.

Respiratory failure is the main threat to life. It arises from ventilatory paralysis, and is exacerbated by excessive bronchial secretions and pulmonary oedema. Assisted ventilation is needed in an intensive care unit. Muscarinic effects of the cholinergic block with salivation, sweating, lacrimation, miosis, hypotension, bradycardia, diarrhoea, tenesmus and faecal incontinence may occur. These complications should be treated with atropine 2 mg i.v., repeated every 5–10 min until there is improvement. The bradycardia is the most easily assessed parameter of improvement.

Pralidoxime is an oxime which functions to partially re-activate the inhibited cholinesterases. It should be given as early as possible in an initial dose of 1 g i.v. which may be repeated in 20 min if there is no improvement. It reduces the nicotinic effects of the poisoning resulting in increased muscle power and decreased fasciculation. Some improvement in the central effects, the confusion, ataxia, drowsiness and seizures, should also be sought. There are no serious adverse effects of pralidoxime. As vomiting may occur early in organophosphate poisoning fluids may need to be replaced.

Recovery occurs very slowly over many weeks. A biochemical measure of improvement is seen in the activity of blood cholinesterases.

NECROTISING VASCULITIS

This term covers a group of conditions in which immunologically determined inflammatory changes and ischaemia occur. Vasculitis with marked inflammatory changes may affect the peripheral nerves, the vascular supply of muscles, and the central nervous system in polyarteritis nodosa. Circulating immune complexes are high in systemic lupus erythematosus (SLE), and also in polyarteritis nodosa and rheumatoid arthritis. In contrast, in Wegener's granulomatosis, chronic inflammatory cell infiltration is the dominant feature, without immune complex deposition. Cranial arteritis and hypersensitivity angiitis are included in this group of disorders.

When acute SLE, polyarteritis nodosa, cranial arteritis or hypersensitivity angiitis involve the nervous system the treatment of choice is steroids. As there is no firm evidence about the optimal starting dose, a wide range has been used between 40 and 100 mg prednisolone daily. A reasonable starting dose is prednisolone 60 mg daily, reducing the total dose in subsequent weeks, according to the patient's clinical response. The ESR is useful but not always a reliable measure of response, particularly in SLE. At the start of treatment there is a small risk that the inflammatory changes affecting the endothelium may result in occlusion of affected vessels, and worsening of symptoms. The other adverse effects are the usual ones with steroid therapy. A steroid psychosis may be difficult to assess in patients with a vasculitis that has already altered mental function. In patients with polyarteritis nodosa which is refractory to conventional oral steroids high doses of 'pulsed' therapy with methylprednisolone have been reported to be successful, without important adverse effects. The methylprednisolone is given in a dose of 30 mg/kg four times in 48 h. The value of steroids in chronic SLE is unclear.

Immunosuppressive drugs, either azathioprine or cyclophosphamide, are alternative or additional drugs. Azathioprine 100–200 mg daily may help with polyarteritis nodosa and hypersensitivity angiitis. Cyclophosphamide is the treatment of choice for Wegener's granulomatosis.

REFERENCES

Forest, J N J, Cox, M, Hong, C, Morrison, G, Bia, M and Singer, I (1978) Superiority of demeclocycline over lithium in the treatment of chronic syndrome of inappropriate secretion of antidiuretic hormone. *New England Journal of Medicine*, **298**, 173–177.

Harper, C (1979) Wernicke's encephalopathy: a more common disease than realised. A neuropathological study of 51 cases. *Journal of Neurology, Neurosurgery and Psychiatry*, **42**, 226–231.

Hartman, D, Rossier, B, Zohlman, R and Schrier, R (1973) Rapid correction of hyponatraemia in the syndrome of inappropriate secretion of antidiuretic hormone. An alternative treatment to hypertonic saline. *Annals of Internal Medicine*, **78**, 870–875.

Lee, K, Moller, L, Hardt, F, Haubek, A and Jensen, E (1979) Alcohol-induced brain damage and liver damage in young males. *Lancet*, **2**, 759–761.

Morgan, M Y, Jakobovits, A W, James, I M and Sherlock, S (1980) Successful use of
bromocriptine in the treatment of chronic hepatic encephalopathy. *Gastro-
enterology*, 78, 663—670.

Victor, M (1970) The role of alcohol in the production of seizures. Epilepsy.
Modern Problems in Pharmacopsychiatry, 4, 185—199.

CHAPTER ELEVEN

Progressive Degenerative Disorders in the Central Nervous System

There are a number of progressive disorders of the nervous system where the aetiology remains unknown and where definitive treatment is not yet possible, others where an infective basis has been defined but where treatment remains unsatisfactory, others which represent an inborn error of metabolism to some extent amenable to biochemical correction, and others which have a genetic basis without a defined biochemical lesion. These conditions have little relation to each other but although individually relatively rare, together they form an important part of neurological practice. Although with some conditions cure is not possible, nevertheless supportive therapy may be of significant help both to the patient and his family in assisting them to cope with an intractable situation. An important group of such disorders is the presenile dementias. Although several of these disorders give rise to particular problems which need to be considered separately the management of dementia provides a situation common to them all and for this reason it is useful to consider these disorders together in a group.

1. PRESENILE DEMENTIA

In this group may be included Alzheimer's and Pick's disease, arteriosclerotic dementia, Jakob—Creutzfeldt disease, progressive supranuclear palsy, certain of the spinocerebellar degenerations such as olivo-ponto-cerebellar degeneration and Huntington's chorea. In Alzheimer's disease there is a progressive falling off of intellectual faculties affecting particularly memory in the early stages, later progressing to the development of signs of focal cerebral impairment such as dysphasia and apraxia. Clinically and pathologically it resembles senile dementia but develops at an earlier age; family studies have shown that cases of Alzheimer's disease rarely develop in close relatives of patients with senile dementia (Larsson *et al.*, 1963). Little is known regarding the aetiology but there is now evidence that the disease affects particularly cholinergic neurones. Pick's disease is relatively rare, the frontal lobes are particularly affected and several patients with the condition not infrequently appear in the same family. Arteriosclerotic dementia differs from Alzheimer and Pick's disease in that the course is episodic rather than continuously progressive and there are frequently associated signs of cerebrovascular insufficiency. In Jakob—Creutzfeldt's disease there is a rapidly progressive dementia associated with progressive paralysis, myoclonic jerking and periodic complexes in the EEG. It has been shown by Gajdusek and Gibbs (1971) to be transmissible to monkeys and it is considered to form one of the group of slow virus infections. Progressive supranuclear palsy or the Steele—Richardson syndrome (Steele *et al.*, 1964) is a condition in which there is paralysis of external ocular movements particularly in the vertical plane associated with Parkinsonian rigidity and dementia, and sometimes also spastic paralysis. The dementia in this condition has been described as a subcortical dementia differing from the dementia seen in conditions such as Alzheimer's disease where there is widespread loss of cortical neurones. In progressive supranuclear palsy slowness of thought is the predominant feature with signs of cortical deficit such as dysphasia being generally absent. The spinocerebellar degenerations which occur in adult life and which are sometimes familial may likewise be associated with dementia as the disease advances. This is particularly so for olivoponto-cerebellar atrophy where Parkinsonian features may also develop. In Huntington's chorea dementia may occur along with the involuntary movements as the disease progresses. This illness provides a particular problem in management in that it is genetically determined, being inherited as an autosomal dominant with nearly complete penetrance. At the present time no method is available for detecting cases before the clinical features have developed. Recent studies of brain material have found reduced levels of γ-aminobutyric acid (GABA) in the basal ganglia and substantia nigra (Perry *et al.*, 1973; Bird *et al.*, 1973).

Management of dementia

In the management of dementia an accurate diagnosis is of paramount importance and there should be no possibility of missing an underlying treatable condition such as a meningioma, subdural haematoma, hypothyroidism, vitamin B_{12} deficiency or a depressive illness in which psychomotor retardation may give a false impression of intellectual impairment. Once a diagnosis has been established important decisions are necessary. The patient himself may not have insight into his disability but responsible relatives must be clearly informed as to the outlook and responsible decisions taken regarding work and employment. If the patient is in a routine job he may be able to continue for a time but work requiring responsibility will have to be given up. In dealing with these problems the services of a professional social worker may be of great value. Ultimately long-term hospital care may become necessary but relatives may be able to manage for a considerable period if adequate steps are taken to enable the patient to cope to a limited extent and measures such as attendance at a day centre or temporary admissions to hospital may do much to alleviate the situation. Whether the patient is at home or in an institution it is important that he should have a stable environment in familiar surroundings and with frequent contact with family and people known to the patient. So far as possible the environment must be organised to maintain the patient's orientation, and occupational therapy should be directed so that the patient is able to attempt and practise tasks which remain within his capacity.

Specific drug therapy has little to offer in the treatment of dementia at the present time. The observation that cholinergic neurones appear to be selectively affected in Alzheimer's disease has led to the use of choline or lecithin since these substances increase acetylcholine in nervous tissue. The value of this treatment is not established. In Jakob—Creutzfeldt disease several case reports have shown improvement following treatment with amantadine (Braham, 1971; Sanders and Dunn, 1973) and in this condition there is a strong case for giving a trial of this drug in a dose of 200—400 mg per day. In arteriosclerotic dementia, and also in Alzheimer's disease and senile dementia, a number of vasodilator substances have been used; with cyclandelate, Hydergine and naftidrofuryl controlled trials have shown a modest improvement (Fine *et al.*, 1970; Young *et al.*, 1974; Gerin, 1969 and 1974). Cyclandelate (Cyclospasmol) is made up in 400 mg tablets and may be given in a dose of three to four tablets a day. Hydergine is a proprietary preparation of ergot alkaloids and is made up in tablets each containing 1.5 mg of co-dergocrine mesylate and it is given in a dose of one tablet three times a day. Naftidrofuryl (Praxilene) is made up in 100 mg capsules and may be given in a dose of one capsule three times a day. In addition to acting as a vasodilator this substance may also have an effect in enhancing cellular metabolism. In general it is not desirable that the patient with dementia should be on a complex regime of medication. Nevertheless medication may be needed to control depression and agitation and if agitation is a problem the phenothiazines are the most satisfactory. Chlormethiazole (Heminevrin) and nitrazepam (Mogadon) are satisfactory preparations for night sedation but it is important to be sure that sleeplessness and restlessness are not caused by intercurrent infection, particularly of the urinary tract, or by joint pains which can be treated by simple analgesics.

Huntington's chorea provides special problems. Phenothiazine drugs are probably the most appropriate for the control of involuntary movements and tetrabenazine is also effective but great care has to be taken in its use in view of the possibility that continuous use may lead to depression. The dementia of Huntington's chorea develops very gradually and insight and memory may be preserved for a long period. Many patients show personality disturbance with psychotic features. Unfortunately, the hereditary nature of the disease imposes severe problems on the family since many of the close relatives of the patient may have to come to terms with the fact that they themselves may later develop the disease or that their children may be affected. At the present time there is no certain means of predicting that a person at risk may develop Huntington's chorea in later life. Changes in the electroencephalogram or in the habituation of the blink reflex do not appear to have predictive value. A significant number of relatives of patients with Huntington's chorea will develop choreiform movements if given levodopa (Klawans *et al.*, 1973) but it is not possible to assess the predictive value of this effect without prolonged follow-up, and the possible psychological effects of a test of this nature when nothing can be done to prevent Huntington's chorea developing in the event of a positive result are daunting.

Motor neurone disease

Motor neurone disease is a progressive disorder of unknown aetiology in which there is progressive wasting of the muscles without sensory disturbance. In some cases when there is also involvement of the long tracts, and if these are involved above the medulla, clinical features of pseudobulbar palsy may develop. Where the long tracts are involved the condition is termed amyotrophic lateral sclerosis; the other two varieties are known as progressive muscular atrophy and progressive bulbar palsy. In addition there is a variety of amyotrophic lateral sclerosis which occurs with a high incidence among the Chamorro population on the island of Guam where it occurs alongside a condition characterised by progressive dementia and Parkinson's disease. The relation of the amyotrophic lateral sclerosis of Guam and the Parkinsonism dementia complex to the motor neurone disease widely encountered in the rest of the world is not understood.

Of the three common varieties of motor neurone disease the most frequently seen is amyotrophic lateral sclerosis which tends to run a steadily progressive course over about 2 years. Progressive bulbar palsy is more rapidly progressive but progressive muscular atrophy may be only slowly progressive with survival extending to 5 years or longer. No method of treatment has been found to have any effect on the natural progress of the disease. Antiviral agents such as amantadine and guanidine (Norris *et al.*, 1974; Norris, 1975) have been tried without any benefit, but Liversedge and Campbell (1974) have found symptomatic relief following the use of pyridostigmine taken along with atropine to reduce the associated production of saliva. Chelating agents such as penicillamine have been used, without benefit, on the suggestion that in some patients the condition may be related to retention in the body of heavy metals such as lead (House *et al.*, 1978). Therefore only symptomatic measures are appropriate and of these amitriptyline may be particularly useful in that it may help to control the depression which often accompanies the disease and also at the same time reduce salivation. Orthopaedic aids may be helpful in controlling foot-drop, and if the patient has difficulty in holding up his head a wheelchair with a head support may be useful. When the patient has difficulty in swallowing, the food should be pulverised with a mixer; if necessary tube feeding may need to be employed. The operation of cricopharyngotomy is sometimes helpful (Loizou *et al.*, 1980). Generally when the patient becomes severely paralysed life expectancy is of limited duration but sometimes, particularly in patients with progressive muscular atrophy, the patient may survive for long periods with virtually no movement in the limbs and in this situation aids such as a possum device may succeed in making the patient's life more tolerable. In general the patient's mind remains clear to the end, and to sustain the patient in this situation is a major challenge to doctor, nursing staff and relatives.

Friedreich's ataxia

This condition is one of a large group of hereditary ataxic disorders which occur in childhood. Other varieties are hereditary spastic paraplegia, peroneal muscular atrophy (Charcot–Marie–Tooth disease) and the Roussy–Levy syndrome. In all these conditions there may be progressive wasting and weakness of the muscles of the lower limbs with difficulty in walking; often there is a pes cavus deformity. In Friedreich's ataxia the symptoms start in childhood and the condition is steadily progressive, but the progress is extremely variable. Some patients become chair-bound before they reach adult life but life expectancy may extend into middle age. Sometimes there are associated abnormalities such as deafness, retinitis pigmentosa and optic atrophy, and the patient may sometimes need to be treated as a partially sighted person. If there is marked deformity of the feet orthopaedic treatment may be necessary but in general management is directed towards keeping the patient as mobile as possible. Aids and appliances such as wheelchairs may be necessary as the child grows older. Friedreich's ataxia is generally inherited as an autosomal recessive but in some families the condition has a dominant inheritance and a careful family history is necessary if appropriate genetic counselling is to be given. Peroneal muscular atrophy, on the other hand, is generally inherited as an autosomal dominant but has a very much more benign course, disability usually remaining slight throughout the greater portion of the patient's life and it may be associated with a normal life expectancy. In this condition genetic counselling may be difficult because subclinical cases occur in which there is no evident deformity or only a mild degree of pes cavus; in some of these patients nerve conduction velocity may be slow and electrophysiological studies are therefore helpful in detecting clinically normal heterozygotes.

Hepatolenticular degeneration (Wilson's disease)

In this condition an excess of copper is absorbed which accumulates in the brain, the liver and other tissues of the body, and there is an increased excretion of copper in the urine. There is a decrease in the serum caeruloplasmin which is the globulin fraction of the serum protein to which the greater part of serum copper is bound. The neurological disturbance is due to changes in the basal ganglia and cavitation in the putamen, globus pallidus and caudate nucleus may be present. Cirrhosis of the liver develops and in the kidneys there may be damage to the proximal renal tubules with excretion in the urine of amino acids, uric acid and calcium. It is inherited as an autosomal recessive and there is a high consanguinity rate among parents.

The aim of treatment is to decrease the total body content of copper. This can be done by giving a low copper diet, avoiding such items as chocolate, mushrooms, dried fruits, shellfish, liver, cocoa, nuts and whisky but the most effective treatment is to use the chelating agent penicillamine which may be given in a dose of 1—2 g per day by mouth. This drug is well tolerated in patients with Wilson's disease but serious side-effects can occur such as the nephrotic syndrome and a lupus-like disease and also thrombocytopenia, granulocytopenia, skin changes and loss of taste. These changes develop less frequently in Wilson's disease than when the drug is used for the treatment of cystinuria or rheumatoid arthritis, possibly because the act of chelation of copper blocks the sulphydryl group on the amino acid to prevent it combining to form antigens with other body proteins. However, if side-effects develop it may be necessary to use BAL (2,3-dimercaptopropanol) in a dose of 2.5 mg/kg body-weight twice daily for 5 days followed by 2 days' rest and continued in successive courses. This drug, however, has to be given by injection so that patients do not readily tolerate it over long periods. Another drug which has been used is tri-ethylene tetramine hydrochloride which seems to be effective and relatively free of side-effects (Walshe, 1973).

Treatment of Wilson's disease is very effective if the condition is recognised early, and many of the neurological features can be reversed by continued therapy. When giving penicillamine it is important to give in addition pyridoxine 50 mg daily as pyridoxine deficiency can result from penicillamine treatment.

When a patient has been identified as suffering from Wilson's disease it is important to examine the other members of the family, in particular the siblings, as these other members of the family — although clinically normal — may have an increased urinary copper or a low caeruloplasmin. If necessary the diagnosis may be confirmed by liver biopsy, and treatment at this stage will have an excellent prospect of preventing the clinical disease developing. It is also possible to identify heterozygotes by finding a low serum caeruloplasmin in association with a normal level of hepatic copper (Bearn, 1972).

REFERENCES

Bearn, A G (1972) Wilson's disease. In: *The Metabolic Basis of Inherited Disease*, 3rd edn, pp. 1033—1050. (Eds) S B Stanbury, J B Wyngaarden and D S Frederickson. McGraw-Hill, New York.

Bird, E D, MacKay, A V P, Rayner, C N and Iversen, L L (1973) Reduced glutamic-acid-decarboxylase activity of post-mortem brain in Huntington's chorea. *Lancet*, 1, 1090—1092.

Braham, J (1971) Jakob—Creutzfeldt disease: treatment by amantadine. *British Medical Journal*, 4, 212—213.

Fine, E W, Lewis, D, Villa-Landa, I and Blakemore, C B (1970) The effect of cyclandelate on mental function in patients with arteriosclerotic brain disease. *British Journal of Psychiatry*, 117, 157—161.

Gajdusek, D C and Gibbs, C J (1971) Transmission of two subacute spongiform encephalopathies of man (Kuru and Creutzfeldt—Jakob disease) to New World monkeys. *Nature*, 230, 588—591.

Gerin, J (1969) Symptomatic treatment of cerebrovascular insufficiency with Hydergine. *Current Therapeutic Research*, **11**, 539–546.

Gerin, J (1974) Double blind trial of naftidrofuryl in the treatment of cerebral arteriosclerosis. *British Journal of Clinical Practice*, **28**, 177–178.

House, A O, Abbott, R J, Davidson, D L W, Ferguson, I T and Lenman, J A R (1978) Response to penicillamine of lead concentrations in CSF and blood in patients with motor neurone disease. *British Medical Journal*, **2**, 1684.

Klawans, H L, Paulson, G W, Ringel, S P and Barbeau, A (1973) The use of L-dopa in the presymptomatic detection of Huntington's chorea. In: *Advances in Neurology*, vol. 1, *Huntington's chorea 1872–1972*, pp. 295–300. (Eds) A Barbeau, T N Chase and G W Paulson. Raven Press, New York.

Larsson, T, Sjögren, T and Jacobson, G (1963) Senile dementia: a clinical, socio-medical and genetic study. *Acta Psychiatrica Scandinavica (Suppl.)*, **167**, 1–259.

Liversedge, L A and Campbell, M J (1974) Motor neurone diseases. In: *Disorders of Voluntary Muscle*, 3rd edn, pp. 775–803. (Ed) J N Walton. Churchill Livingstone, Edinburgh.

Loizou, L A, Small, M and Dalton, G A (1980) Cricopharyngeal myotomy in motor neurone disease. *Journal of Neurology, Neurosurgery and Psychiatry*, **43**, 42–45.

Norris, F H (1975) Adult spinal motor neurone disease. Progressive muscular atrophy (Aran's disease) in relation to amyotrophic lateral sclerosis. In: *Handbook of Clinical Neurology*, vol. 22, *System Disorders and Atrophies*, Part II, pp. 1–56. (Eds) P J Vinken and G W Bruyn in collaboration with J M B V De Jong. North Holland Publishing Co., Amsterdam.

Norris, F H Jr, Calanchini, P R, Fallat, R J, Sandra Panchari, R P T and Jewett, B (1974) The administration of guanidine in amyotrophic lateral sclerosis. *Neurology (Minneapolis)*, **24**, 721–728.

Perry, T L, Hansen, S and Kloster, M (1973) Huntington's chorea: deficiency of gamma-aminobutyric acid in the brain. *New England Journal of Medicine*, **288**, 337–342.

Sanders, W L and Dunn, T L (1973) Creutzfeldt–Jakob disease treated with amantadine. *Journal of Neurology, Neurosurgery and Psychiatry*, **36**, 581–584.

Steele, J C, Richardson, J C and Olszewski, J (1964) Progressive supranuclear palsy. *Archives of Neurology*, **10**, 333–359.

Walshe, J M (1973) Copper chelation in patients with Wilson's disease, A comparison of penicillamine and triethylene tetramine dihydrochloride. *Quarterly Journal of Medicine*, N.S. **42**, 441–452.

Young, J, Hall, P and Blakemore, C (1974) Treatment of the cerebral manifestations of arteriosclerosis with cyclandelate. *British Journal of Psychiatry*, **124**, 177–180.

CHAPTER TWELVE

Disorders of Peripheral Nerves

The function of peripheral nerves can be affected directly by trauma, local pressure or by a wide variety of inflammatory, metabolic, deficiency or toxic disorders. Accurate diagnosis is important if specific therapy is to be applied, but in a substantial proportion of patients with peripheral neuropathy the cause cannot be determined and treatment depends on the application of appropriate symptomatic measures. In this chapter consideration will be given to describing the treatment applicable to the principal varieties of peripheral nerve lesion or neuropathy and this will be followed by an account of the general measures which are available for restoration of function.

NERVE TRAUMA AND NERVE ENTRAPMENT

Nerve trauma may take the form of acute section of a peripheral nerve or contusion such as may arise from an acute injury, or may result from local pressure from neighbouring tissues. In certain situations, such as the spiral groove of the humerus where the radial nerve is vulnerable or the head of the fibula where the common peroneal nerve may be affected, peripheral nerves can be readily damaged by fracture and the brachial plexus may be injured by traction injuries, in the severest form of which the roots are avulsed from the spinal cord. Where continued local pressure occurs on a nerve at a particular site this gives rise to an entrapment neuropathy. Thus compression of the median nerve as it passes through the carpal tunnel at the wrist gives rise to the carpal tunnel syndrome but entrapment can occur at many different sites and these will be considered in the section dealing with individual peripheral nerves.

Traumatic lesions of peripheral nerves have been considered in great detail by Seddon (1975) and by Sunderland (1978). Seddon (1943) has classified peripheral nerve injury according to whether the damage gives rise to a temporary conduction block or causes destruction of the axon at the site of injury leading to Wallerian degeneration. Conduction block with preservation of the axon is described as neurapraxia; where the axon is damaged but the connective tissue of the nerve is preserved the lesion is defined as axonotmesis. Neurotmesis is where the whole thickness of the nerve including the connective tissue is divided. Sunderland (1978) classifies nerve injury into five degrees of increasing severity. First- and second-degree injury correspond with neurapraxia and axonotmesis respectively, and fifth-degree injury corresponds with neurotmesis. In third-degree injury, in addition to axonol damage and Wallerian degeneration, there is disorganisation of the internal structure of the funiculi and in fourth-degree injury this damage to the connective tissue structure of the nerve is so severe that continuity of the funiculi is lost.

These distinctions are important clinically as well as being of pathological interest. In neurapraxia recovery is generally rapid but following axonotmesis and neurotmesis recovery can only take place by regeneration. In neurotmesis nerve suture will be necessary if recovery is to take place, and in fourth-degree injury useful spontaneous recovery seldom occurs and surgical repair of the nerve with excision of thc involved segment is generally necessary. The regrowth of the regenerating axon takes place at a rate of about 3.0 mm per day but there may be a latent period of several weeks before regeneration starts, depending on the nature of the lesion and the amount of fibrous tissue; there may also be a further delay between re-innervation and functional recovery.

If it seems likely that the effect of injury has been to interrupt the anatomical continuity of the nerve then it is advisable surgically to explore the nerve. This should be undertaken if the injury is due to a penetrating wound or if the lesion is in a proximal part of the nerve. With a lesion in a distal part of the nerve it may be reasonable to delay exploration for 3—4 weeks when evidence of regeneration would be expected. With penetrating wounds if the wound is clean it may be appropriate to suture the nerve as soon as possible after the injury — primary suture. This is perhaps particularly important in situations such as the hand where it may be difficult to identify the damaged nerves after an interval of time. Where the wound is extensive, however, primary suture may be difficult and it is generally preferable after primary treatment of the wound to leave an interval of 1—4 weeks before carrying out secondary suture.

GENERALISED NEUROPATHIES

General metabolic disease

Diabetes mellitus

The commonest neuropathy in diabetes is a distal symmetrical, predominantly sensory, polyneuropathy but other varieties include proximal mononeuropathies, cranial nerve palsies and a symmetrical autonomic neuropathy. Proximal mononeuropathy often involves the femoral nerve, and muscle-wasting resulting from this lesion is a common presentation of diabetic amyotrophy. Segmental demyelination is frequently present in affected nerves and this is generally considered to be due to a metabolic process affecting the Schwann cells (Thomas and Lascelles, 1965) but ischaemic changes including infarcts may be seen in peripheral nerves, particularly in diabetic mononeuropathy (Raff et al., 1968). Although in many cases of diabetic neuropathy symptoms present at times when the diabetes is poorly controlled, in other patients the neuropathy may be the first symptom of diabetes and in others it may seem to progress in spite of careful control of the blood sugar levels. Nevertheless, scrupulous control of the diabetic state is particularly important whenever diabetic neuropathy is recognised and Bruyn and Garland (1970) emphasise the improvement which may take place in diabetic amyotrophy if the blood sugar is maintained within the physiological range. In sensory neuropathy great care must be taken of the feet, which are readily injured by minor trauma; carbamazepine is sometimes effective in relieving the pain. In diabetes peripheral nerves may be vulnerable to entrapment and local decompression may be advisable when this occurs. The treatment of autonomic neuropathy is considered at the end of this chapter.

Uraemic neuropathy

The neuropathy of patients with uraemia is a predominantly sensory neuropathy and symptoms include unpleasant paraesthesiae, restless legs and the symptoms tend to spread proximally from the feet. The symptoms are only partially relieved by renal dialysis but generally remit following renal transplantation.

The neuropathy of hepatic failure

A mixed sensorimotor neuropathy may occur in patients with hepatic disease. How far this is due to effects of coincident alcoholism or diabetes is uncertain but neuropathy may be a feature also in primary biliary cirrhosis, and a polyneuropathy which is sometimes seen in acute hepatitis may be a variant of the Guillain—Barré syndrome. Other neuropathies seen in liver disease would appear not to be a single entity, and treatment should be directed to correction of the particular metabolic disturbance such as, for example, vitamin B deficiency in alcoholic cirrhosis.

Thyroid disease

Entrapment neuropathies such as carpal tunnel syndrome may occur in myxoedema (Murray and Simpson, 1958) but a symmetrical polyneuropathy is occasionally seen in hypothyroidism.

Carcinoma

Among the neurological non-metastatic manifestations which may be associated with carcinoma a relatively common variety is a sensorimotor peripheral neuropathy (Brain, Croft and Wilkinson, 1969). Little is known regarding the effects of treatment of the primary neoplastic condition on this type of neuropathy, and its particular importance lies in the recognition that an occult carcinoma may be present in a patient who presents with a neuropathy without evident cause. A motor neurone disease-like syndrome is sometimes seen in association with carcinoma and this has been reported to improve following treatment of the primary condition (Mitchell and Olczak, 1979).

Acute intermittent porphyria (*see* Chapter 10)

Peripheral neuropathy may occur in acute intermittent porphyria and the clinical features have been reviewed by Ridley (1969). The condition is inherited as an autosomal dominant with incomplete penetrance so genetic advice may be indicated for affected relatives. Episodes of acute porphyria may sometimes be provoked by exposure to alcohol, barbiturates or sulphonamides and great care should be taken in the use of drugs with affected patients. The neuropathy may be acute and severe with paralysis of the respiratory and bulbar muscles, and in these cases artificial ventilation with tracheostomy may be necessary.

Connective tissue disorders

Peripheral neuropathy occurs quite commonly in polyarteritis nodosa

(Bleehen *et al.*, 1963) and in a smaller proportion of cases of systemic lupus erythematosus (SLE) (Johnson and Richardson, 1968). In either condition it may take the form of mononeuritis multiplex. Polyarteritis, regardless of whether peripheral neuropathy is present or not, generally requires treatment with steroids or other immuno-suppressants. In SLE peripheral neuropathy is much less common than central nervous system manifestations but improvement has followed treatment with steroids (Gargour *et al.*, 1964). In rheumatoid arthritis entrapment neuropathies are a common occurrence which may be relieved by surgical decompression or local injection of hydrocortisone. Some patients have a distal sensory polyneuropathy affecting the lower limbs which is associated with slowing of nerve conduction velocity; this neuropathy may be aggravated by corticosteroids (Ferguson and Slocumb, 1961). In a further variety there may be a sensory motor neuropathy affecting the upper and lower limbs with normal nerve conduction velocity, and in this variety penicillamine may be of value (Golding, 1973) and cytotoxic immunosuppressive agents may be given (Bradley, 1974).

INFECTION

Diphtheria

The infective agent of diphtheria produces a neurotoxin which causes demyelination of peripheral nerves. There is usually a latent period between the development of pharyngitis and the nerve damage which may be sometimes as long as 3 weeks. When it occurs it may cause first a palatal palsy and then a bulbar palsy with widespread peripheral neuropathy. Tracheostomy and artificial ventilation may be necessary. Antitoxin probably has little effect on the neuropathy once it is established but remyelination with recovery of paralysis generally occurs if the patient survives.

Leprosy

In this condition there is predominant involvement of cutaneous nerves with severe anaesthesia giving rise to local trauma. In *lepromatous leprosy* hypertrophic skin lesions occur and *Mycobacterium leprae* is found in the peripheral nerves. The immune response is humoral with an elevated serum immunoglobulin, enlarged lymph nodes and a negative lepromin skin test. The neuropathy is generally distal and predominantly sensory. In *tuberculoid leprosy* there is atrophy and depigmentation of the skin, and neuropathic phenomena are prominent. The immune response is cellular and the lepromin skin test is positive. Polyneuritis multiplex occurs with nodular thickening of the peripheral nerves.

Lepromatous leprosy runs a steadily progressive and, in the absence of treatment, generally fatal course. Tuberculoid leprosy, on the other hand, runs a relatively protracted course with remissions and relapses; mild cases may recover completely even without treatment. The most useful drug in the treatment of leprosy is diaminodiphenylsulphone (dapsone) which can be given in a dose of 50—100 mg daily by mouth (1 mg/kg to children). In lepromatous leprosy it may take from 3 to 8 years for all skin lesions to be healed and for acid-fast bacilli no longer to be isolated from the lesions. In tuberculoid leprosy a satisfactory clinical response may be evident after 1 or 2 years. To avoid relapse maintenance therapy should be continued for up to 3 years in tuberculoid leprosy, for 20 years or longer in lepromatous leprosy and for up to 15 years in intermediate forms. Reactions to sulphones are generally not severe but may include polyneuropathy in addition to anaemia, agranulocytosis and psychiatric reactions.

Other drugs which are available include rifampicin, which is bactericidal, clofazimine, thiambutazone and ethionamide. Because it may cause pigmentation of the skin clofazimine is more suitable for treating dark- than light-skinned patients. Because of the possibility of drug resistance it has been recommended to start treatment with dapsone and one other drug such as clofazimine, and where the organism is known to be drug-resistant with a combination of three drugs such as clofazimine, rifampicin and one other drug.

During treatment lepra reactions may occur. These include tender erythematous nodules (erythema nodosum leprosum) and they may be treated with mild analgesics. Corticosteroids may also be helpful but in severe or prolonged reactions clofazimine in a dose of 100 mg every other day increasing to 400 mg daily may be used. Sometimes patients with leprosy develop features such as a claw hand or a foot drop due to peroneal nerve palsy, and treatment of these may require orthopaedic measures. BCG vaccination of children may be of value in prophylaxis.

Acute post-infective polyneuropathy

Patients with this condition who were described by Guillain—Barré and Strohl in 1916 all had a raised protein with normal cell count in the CSF, but this finding is not invariable and some patients have a normal CSF and a few have an elevated cell count with normal protein. In many instances the illness follows a virus infection and commonly it gives rise to both proximal and distal weakness with paraesthesiae and often sensory impairment. Many patients recover completely but a significant number are left with persistent deficit. The pathogenesis has been reviewed by Hughes (1979). In many respects the condition resembles experimental allergic neuropathy produced in animals by injection of peripheral nerve with Freund's adjuvant, and it is possible that cell-mediated immunity to neural antigens is an important factor in the pathogenesis. If viral agents invaded the peripheral nerves to deposit antigen in the Schwann cell this could evoke an immune response. Early studies with corticosteroids suggested that these might be helpful in the treatment of the Guillain—Barré syndrome (Jackson *et al.*, 1957). Several careful studies, however (Löffel *et al.*, 1977; Hughes *et al.*, 1978) have shown no improvement with steroids and in fact the overall effect of steroids in the study of Hughes *et al.* was that improvement was slower in the treated group. Although it has been held that some patients with Guillain—Barré syndrome may improve when given steroids, and relapse if the treatment is withdrawn, it would seem at the present time that there is not adequate evidence to indicate prescribing ACTH or prednisolone in this condition. Treatment therefore remains symptomatic and should include rest in the early stages but with regular physiotherapy and passive movements to the limbs. Great care must be taken to recognise respiratory difficulty and about 10 per cent of patients will require artificial respiration with tracheostomy. Autonomic disturbances sometimes occur and these must be dealt with appropriately (*see* below). In patients who are severely paralysed there is a risk that deep vein thrombosis may develop and consideration should be given to the advisability of prophylactic therapy with heparin. As with steroid therapy the place of immunosuppressive therapy with azathioprine or cyclophosphamide remains uncertain and a number of studies have shown conflicting results (Yuill *et al.*, 1970; Rosen and Vastola, 1976).

Chronic relapsing polyneuropathy

In this neuropathy involvement is predominantly motor and the initial episode may be very similar to the Guillain—Barré syndrome with an elevated CSF protein and slowing of nerve conduction velocity. In this condition there may be a striking response to corticosteroid therapy, with reductions in dosage being accompanied by relapse, and improvement occurring again as the dose is increased (Austin, 1958; Thomas *et al.*, 1969). Either ACTH or prednisolone may be effective. Bradley

(1974) recommends giving a dose of corticosteroid adequate to suppress the condition over a period of several months and then only reducing by a very small amount — perhaps by 5 mg of prednisolone every month. If the condition relapses as the dose is reduced it will need to be increased again, but sometimes the steroid therapy may be eventually withdrawn completely.

Neuralgic amyotrophy

In this condition the brachial plexus is generally affected, usually on one side, but sometimes it may involve only a single cord or peripheral nerve. Early cases were described during the Second World War by Parsonage and Turner (1948) and episodes may follow an infection, an operation or trauma, or the administration of a vaccine; an allergic mechanism has been postulated. Initially, there is severe pain and this is followed by weakness and sometimes sensory loss. The long-term prognosis is favourable but improvement may not be evident for several months and may not be complete for 2 or more years. Some patients are left with residual weakness. In the acute stage analgesics are indicated to relieve the pain and corticosteroids may bring symptomatic relief but they do not appear to have any long-term benefit on the weakness or sensory disturbance.

Hereditary neuropathies

In this group of conditions there is generally little that can be done by way of effective treatment but accurate diagnosis is important because the natural history and prognosis varies widely in the different conditions and it may be important to be able to provide appropriate genetic advice. The disorders include a number of metabolic conditions such as porphyria, which has already been considered, and primary amyloidosis, a group of hypertrophic polyneuropathies including Charcot—Marie—Tooth disease, Refsum's disease and the hypertrophic neuropathy of Dejerine—Sottas, and the spinal muscular atrophies. This latter group is important because in some patients spinal muscular atrophy can readily be confused with muscular dystrophy. Refsum's disease is of particular interest because it has been found to be associated with a metabolic defect in which phytanic acid (3,7,11,15-tetramethyl-hexadecanoic acid) is found in the blood and tissues of the body; the condition can be relieved by a diet lacking in dairy fats and green produce and with a low phytol content (Steinberg et al., 1970). In Charcot—Marie—Tooth disease or peroneal muscular atrophy inheritance is as an autosomal dominant and clinically healthy heterozygotes can sometimes be recognised by finding a marked slowing of nerve conduction velocity. The principal varieties of hereditary neuropathy and their usual mode of inheritance are shown in Table 12.1.

Vitamin deficiency

Deficiency of vitamin B_1 or thiamine, if severe, gives rise to beri-beri where damage to peripheral nerves results in the dry form and damage to the heart with congestive failure gives rise to the wet form. Thiamine is the coenzyme for three enzymes; namely, pyruvate decarboxylase, α-ketobutyrate decarboxylase and transketolase, all of which are necessary in carbohydrate metabolism with deficiency leading to failure of breakdown of pyruvate and lactate, which accumulate. The hypothalamic region and brainstem may also be affected giving rise to Wernicke's encephalopathy which is a confusional state with ophthalmoplegia, loss of memory and confabulation (Korsakoff's syndrome). Beri-beri may occur in the tropics in people living on a diet of polished rice, but thiamine deficiency may also be one factor in the neuropathy of

Table 12.1   The hereditary neuropathies

Spinal muscular atrophy
   Proximal
      Infantile (Werdnig—Hoffmann) — autosomal recessive
      Juvenile (Kugelberg Welander) — autosomal recessive
      Adult — autosomal recessive or dominant or X-linked recessive
   Distal — autosomal recessive or dominant
   Juvenile progressive bulbar palsy (Fazio—Londe) — autosomal recessive
   Scapuloperoneal — autosomal dominant, rarely recessive

Hypertrophic polyneuropathies
   Peroneal muscular atrophy (Charcot—Marie—Tooth) — autosomal dominant, rarely recessive
   Hypertrophic neuropathy (Dejerine—Sottas) — autosomal dominant
   Refsum's disease — autosomal recessive

Peroneal muscular atrophy, neuronal type — autosomal dominant

Familial amyloidosis — autosomal dominant

Hereditary sensory radicular neuropathy — autosomal dominant

---

alcoholism and the neuropathies which may follow partial gastrectomy or develop in association with a malabsorption syndrome. Thiamine can be administered by mouth or by intramuscular injection in a dose of 50 or 100 mg per day, but where a neuropathy is associated with vitamin deficiency other vitamins may also be lacking. It is then advisable to supplement therapy with thiamine with pyridoxine 100 mg, riboflavine, 5 mg, and nicotinamide in a dose of 200 mg. These substances can all be given either by mouth or by i.m. injection.

Vitamin B_{12} is necessary both for haemopoiesis and the integrity of nerve tissue. If there is deficiency there may be peripheral neuropathy, in addition to changes in the brain and spinal cord, and megaloblastic anaemia. Deficiency occurs in pernicious anaemia when there is loss of gastric intrinsic factor; it can also occur in a variety of malabsorption syndromes and as a result of dietary deficiency. The peripheral neuropathy will generally respond rapidly to i.m. hydroxycobalamin (vitamin B_{12}) in a dose of 1000 μg per day.

The neuropathies which occur in association with adult coeliac disease (Cooke and Smith, 1966) and following partial gastrectomy (Banerji and Hurwitz, 1971) may each be associated with multiple vitamin deficiencies including vitamin B_{12}, but not every case will respond fully to vitamin replacement therapy.

Other vitamin deficiencies occurring in isolation are rare, but nicotinic acid deficiency gives rise to pellagra and riboflavine deficiency may be associated with a 'burning-feet' syndrome. Deficiency of pyridoxine gives rise to a distal sensory neuropathy; this variety of neuropathy may result from treatment with isoniazid which may interfere with the metabolism of pyridoxine.

Toxic neuropathy

A wide variety of drugs and other chemicals can give rise to toxic neuropathy. The most important aspect of the treatment of toxic neuropathy is its recognition, so that exposure to the offending substance can be withdrawn, but in a number of instances other supplementary measures are helpful. Thus in alcoholic neuropathy — which may be associated with a 'burning-feet' syndrome. Deficiency of pyrisystem but which is frequently associated with vitamin deficiencies — correction of the nutritional deficiency may also be helpful. In the neuropathy due to isoniazid — which is due to interference with pyridoxine metabolism — the condition can be effectively treated by taking pyridoxine. In neuropathy due to heavy metals such as lead, chelating agents which may mobilise and remove the offending substance from the body may also be helpful. Examples of some of the substances which may give rise to toxic neuropathy are shown in Table 12.2 (*see* also Appendix).

Restless legs

This condition, in which unpleasant creeping sensations occur in the legs particularly when they are at rest and at night, was described in detail by Ekbom in 1944 who has reviewed the clinical features and management (Ekbom, 1970). It is probably not correct to speak of the condition as a peripheral neuropathy since the creeping sensations are different from the paraesthesiae commonly experienced with peripheral nerve involvement and the condition is not accompanied by any physical signs of neurological involvement. There is a strong association with anaemia, particularly due to iron deficiency, and it is important both to examine the blood and to estimate the serum iron as correction of iron deficiency may relieve the symptoms without other treatment. Some patients respond to vasodilators such as tolazoline hydrochloride (Priscol) which is made up in 25 mg tablets which can be taken in an initial dose of half a tablet once or twice daily, or nicotinyl alcohol (Ronicol) which is made up in 25 mg tablets which can be taken in a dose of one or two tablets three or four times a day. Probably the most useful single symptomatic remedy is diazepam taken in the evening, sometimes along with a mild analgesic such as aspirin or paracetamol. Other patients will respond to carbamazepine, and chlorpromazine may

Table 12.2   Toxins which may give rise to neuropathy

Drugs	*Industrial chemicals*
Nitrofurantoin	Arsenic
Isoniazid	Carbon tetrachloride
Phenytoin	Glue
Vincristine	Acrylamide
Disulfiram	Triorthocresyl phosphate
Chloroquine	
Heavy metals	
Lead	
Mercury	
Thallium	
Gold	

be helpful although the symptom of akathisia which sometimes occurs as a side-effect of phenothiazine derivatives in large doses may closely resemble the syndrome of restless legs.

Sarcoidosis

Involvement of the nervous system occurs in about 5 per cent of patients with sarcoidosis and the brain and spinal cord, also the meninges, nerve roots, peripheral nerves and cranial nerves can be affected. The peripheral neuropathy is characteristically a multiple mononeuropathy (mononeuritis multiplex). The facial nerves are frequently involved, sometimes bilaterally, and the facial palsy frequently recovers rapidly. Peripheral nerve involvement may, however, run a chronic course and meningeal and central nervous system involvement may run a progressive and sometimes fatal course.

In general the course of sarcoidosis is benign, many patients remitting spontaneously; probably less than a third of patients with sarcoidosis require treatment. With progressive lesions, however, steroid therapy can be indicated and may be effective in moderate dosage. The neurological features of sarcoid have been reviewed by Matthews (1975).

MONONEUROPATHIES

Cranial nerves

In general the importance of cranial nerve lesions lies in their diagnostic significance as symptoms of a possibly treatable disorder of the nervous system. Thus lesions of the motor nerves to the eye may be associated with raised intracranial pressure or to a space-occupying lesion, such as a tumour or an aneurysm, or be due to a demyelinating disorder, to myasthenia gravis or to diabetes; in each of these conditions treatment is that of the primary disorder. Symptomatic treatment of an ocular palsy may include covering one eye to avoid diplopia, or surgical treatment to correct a squint or relieve ptosis. Pain may arise in the distribution of the trigeminal nerve and the glossopharyngeal nerve; this is discussed in Chapter 5. The 7th or facial nerve is particularly susceptible to inflammation or injury and is considered in greater detail.

The facial nerve

Bell's palsy is the commonest affection of the facial nerve. Usually it is an isolated neuropathy which develops without evident cause in a healthy person. Facial palsy, however, is sometimes associated with herpes zoster affecting the geniculate ganglion when there may be vesicles in the internal auditory meatus and the soft palate and sometimes loss of taste sensation and deafness. Facial palsy can also occur in post-infective polyneuritis and as an occasional feature in multiple sclerosis.

In Bell's palsy more than half the patients make a complete recovery, often within the course of a few weeks; but in about 40 per cent there is some degree of denervation and in these patients recovery may be delayed and is often incomplete. In a small number, possibly about 15 per cent, denervation is severe and the patient may be left with no useful recovery (Taverner, 1959). In the clinical assessment of the patient severe pain in the region of the ear, and absence of taste on the affected side, are sometimes taken as unfavourable prognostic signs; whereas if the facial palsy is incomplete a few days after it has developed this is generally associated with a good recovery. Electrodiagnostic techniques are also helpful in assessing the prognosis as evidence of severe or partial denervation may suggest that recovery will be slow and incomplete. Nerve conduction measurement to demonstrate either a delayed or absent evoked response after stimulating the facial nerve at the angle of the jaw may be particularly helpful. In the management of facial palsy probably the most important aim is to prevent the continuity of the facial nerve being interrupted by compression within the facial canal. For this reason surgical decompression has been advocated but probably the most effective measure is to administer corticosteroids as early as possible after the facial palsy has developed. This can be given as corticotrophin but it may be more effective to give prednisolone in an initial dose of 30–50 mg per day given in diminishing doses over a period of 10 days to a fortnight (Taverner *et al.*, 1971). If the facial palsy is severe, with inability to close the eye and no movement of the affected side of the mouth, it is important to protect the eye from injury and also to prevent contractures developing on the paralysed side of the face. To protect the eye it may be necessary to perform a tarsorrhaphy and to protect the face from contracture the patient should be instructed to carry out regular passive movements of the face in front of a mirror. It may also be helpful to apply a dental splint to maintain the position of the angle of the mouth. This can be attached to one of the teeth and it is important that it should be checked from time to time as too much tension on the splint can also give rise to contracture. Electrical treatment also has its advocates but while it may prevent muscle-wasting taking place it has no effect on the rate of regeneration (*see* below).

Recurrent episodes of facial palsy occur in some patients. Generally no cause for this is discovered and each episode is treated appropriately as if it were an isolated episode. In the *Melkersson—Rosenthal syndrome* episodes of recurrent facial paralysis occur in association with swelling of the lips and face and fissuring of the tongue. The natural course of the illness is variable but recurrent episodes may lead to varying degrees of facial paralysis and coarsening of the features. The most effective treatment is corticosteroids given as early as possible after the onset of an episode. Hornstein (1970) recommends prednisolone in an initial dose of 40—50 mg per day, continuing for at least 2 weeks but sometimes for longer.

The facial nerve is readily damaged by fractures of the temporal bone and in traumatic lesions of this kind electrical testing to establish the continuity of the facial nerve may be of value in deciding whether and at what time surgical exploration may be indicated.

Clonic facial hemispasm is an intractable and progressive condition which usually occurs apparently spontaneously, although it may be a sequel occasionally to a previous facial palsy (*see* Chapter 5).

The median nerve

Injury to the median nerve is most likely to take place at the wrist, as for example following a Colles' fracture, but it may also be injured at the elbow and compression or entrapment of the nerve may take place either in the carpal tunnel or at the elbow where it passes between the two heads of pronator teres. In the carpal tunnel syndrome there are sometimes predisposing factors such as pregnancy, myxoedema, rheumatoid arthritis or diabetes, and nerve conduction studies are useful not only to demonstrate a local lesion of the median nerve at this site but also to rule out a more widespread neuropathy. Temporary relief in mild cases may sometimes be obtained by the application of night splints and by injection of hydrocortisone into the carpal tunnel, sometimes supplemented by diuretics. Definitive treatment, however, requires surgical decompression by division of the carpal ligament. In the pronator teres syndrome surgical decompression is likewise effective.

The ulnar nerve

Compression of the ulnar nerve may occur at the elbow where it may be entrapped by the origin of flexor carpi ulnaris (Osborne, 1959) and where its superficial situation renders it vulnerable to local pressure; in this situation the nerve can be readily stretched against the ulnar groove if there is a valgus deformity resulting from fractures near the elbow. Treatment is by anterior transposition of the ulnar nerve and Osborne (1959) has advocated an operation in which a longitudinal division is made of the aponeurotic covering which fills the gap between the two heads of flexor carpi ulnaris. Injury to the ulnar nerve may also occur as it enters the hand at the wrist, and in the hand the deep branch of the ulnar nerve may be affected giving rise to weakness of the intrinsic muscles of the hand without sensory impairment. In either instance there is frequently a history of trauma and surgical exploration of the hand will often show a ganglion in relation to the nerve. Frequently, however, spontaneous improvement takes place and Seddon (1975) recommends a conservative approach with a period of rest before exploration of the nerve is considered.

The radial nerve

The radial nerve is most vulnerable to injury in the spiral groove where it may be injured by fracture of the humerus or by local pressure as in 'Saturday night palsy'. The posterior interosseous nerve may likewise be injured as it passes through the supinator muscle when it may be pressed on by a variety of innocent swellings such as ganglia, lipomata or by post-traumatic fibrosis. The Saturday night palsy generally recovers spontaneously with conservative therapy; with a posterior interosseous palsy it may be difficult to establish the cause on clinical grounds and exploration is sometimes advisable.

Thoracic outlet syndrome

In this condition the lower trunk of the brachial plexus and sometimes the subclavian artery may be compressed between the scalenus anticus muscle and a cervical rib or a fibrous band. In severe cases there is pain in the arm, weakness of the intrinsic muscles of the hand with paraesthesiae in the ulnar distribution and sometimes a cold hand with hyperhydrosis. The vasomotor changes are not always present and mild cases frequently respond favourably to conservative measures. Transfer to a lighter occupation and the wearing of a sling may be helpful but probably the most useful single measure is the prescription of remedial exercises to improve the posture of the patient and the strength of the shoulder girdle muscles. In severe cases surgical treatment with exploration of the area and removal of a cervical rib may be advisable.

Common peroneal nerve

This nerve is vulnerable to pressure as it winds round the neck of the fibula. Entrapment may also take place under the tendinous arch of origin of the peroneus longus and this may be treated by surgical decompression (Sidey, 1969). With local compression lesions recovery generally takes place when the pressure is relieved but an orthotic support may be necessary to correct the foot-drop during the period of recovery.

The femoral nerve

The femoral nerve is derived from segments L.2, 3 and 4 and lesions of the femoral nerve may be difficult to distinguish from lesions of the lumbar plexus. A mononeuritis affecting the femoral nerve may occur in diabetes but Biemond (1970) describes an idiopathic femoral neuropathy for which no cause has so far been found but which may be due to a reversible ischaemic lesion. The prognosis is favourable, complete recovery usually taking place from a few weeks to several months, and helpful symptomatic treatment includes temporary bed rest and the local application of warmth, in particular short-wave irradiation, above the groin.

The posterior tibial nerve

Entrapment of the posterior tibial nerve may occur where it enters the foot close to the medial malleolus giving rise to pain affecting the toes and the sole of the foot. This syndrome, which closely resembles the carpal tunnel syndrome in the hand, is known as the tarsal tunnel syndrome. It was described by Keck in 1962 and it may be relieved by surgical decompression of the nerve.

Meralgia paraesthetica

In this condition the patient complains of unpleasant sensations in the distribution of the lateral femoral cutaneous nerve which are felt along the outer aspect of the thigh. It may be due to irritation of the nerve where it emerges beneath the inguinal ligament where it is angulated at the anterior superior iliac spine. Stevens (1957), however, has emphasised that the nerve has a long intra-abdominal course also, in which it may be vulnerable to trauma. If a local anaesthetic injected medial to the anterior superior iliac spine relieves the symptom then it is likely to be due to a lesion at the attachment of the inguinal ligament. The course is generally benign with spontaneous remission frequently occurring; probably most cases should be treated conservatively. Surgical treatment includes decompression by cutting the deep inferior fasciculus of the inguinal ligament and resection of the nerve but neither operation guarantees certain relief (Seddon, 1975).

GENERAL MANAGEMENT OF NEUROPATHY

In the earlier sections of this chapter those specific measures which may be helpful in different varieties of peripheral neuropathy have been described. In the present state of knowledge many conditions can only be relieved to a limited extent but appropriate general measures must always be undertaken to preserve function and relieve particular symptoms. For a detailed review of some of the measures at present available the reader is referred to Brown and Opitz (1970).

Muscle weakness

In the treatment of muscle paralysis physiotherapy should be instituted as early as possible. When there is no voluntary movement this should consist of passive movement to prevent stiffness of the joints and lessen any oedema or swelling, and as power improves this must be supplemented by active exercises designed to strengthen and re-educate the affected muscles. Electrical stimulation has been found to delay wasting in denervated muscle (Gutmann and Guttmann, 1944) and this would also appear to be the case with human peripheral nerve injuries (Jackson, 1945). However, it is not certain how far electrotherapy affects the long-term recovery following nerve lesions but Seddon (1975) considers that it has a useful function in the treatment of injuries to nerves supplying the hand. Splinting is important to prevent stretching of paralysed muscles and also to promote useful recovery of function, as for example the simple ortholon splint to correct foot-drop, and cock-up splints to a paralysed hand. 'Lively splints', in which movement is assisted by springs, may aid in promoting the recovery of movement. Occupational therapy is important to enable the patient, by the provision of aids, home adaptations and suitable training, to adapt to the disability. The severely paralysed patient may still retain useful function using electronic devices activated by remote control, such as the possum.

Sensory symptoms

When skin is denervated it is readily injured and if the patient is paralysed great care must be exercised in protecting the skin from pressure and in regular turning of the patient. The severe pain of *causalgia* is fortunately rare. It is most likely to occur after a missile wound giving rise to an incomplete lesion, nearly always in the median or sciatic nerves or in the brachial plexus; it may be due to a false synapse forming between autonomic and somatic fibres in the affected nerve. Injection of a local anaesthetic into the appropriate autonomic ganglia will bring temporary relief, and if this occurs sympathectomy is indicated. More common are so-called irritative lesions or *hyperpathia* in which pain or hypersensitivity of the skin occurs in the situation of the nerve injury, often associated with dryness or moistness of the affected part. Treatment is difficult, but spontaneous improvement or even remission not infrequently occurs. Exploration of the injured nerve is sometimes indicated and resection of part of the nerve may sometimes give relief. Some patients respond to medication with antidepressant drugs.

Autonomic dysfunction

Affection of the autonomic system may lead to severe postural hypotension; it may also affect sweating and the control of the bladder and bowel. In males impotence may be a problem. Although postural hypotension is a particular feature of peripheral neuropathy, particularly diabetic neuropathy, it is also found in Parkinson's disease in association with levodopa therapy and the Shy Drager (1960) syndrome and in familial dysautonomia (Riley *et al.*, 1949). It may be a major problem in patients with transection of the cord above the mid-dorsal level.

Management of postural hypotension is difficult but some patients benefit from sleeping with the head of the bed raised. This may have the effect of increasing the release of renin by reducing the renal arterial pressure. Pooling of blood in the lower part of the body may be reduced by supporting elastic stockings and occasionally inflatable pressure suits may be helpful. Ephedrine up to 25 mg three times daily is sometimes helpful but probably the most useful medication is fludrocortisone 0.1 mg per day, which acts by increasing the sensitivity of the vessels to circulating noradrenaline. Current practice has been reviewed by Bannister (1979).

Cholinergic drugs such as bethanecol chloride and distigmine bromide may assist in bladder-emptying. Constipation may be a problem leading to faecal impaction, and the addition of softening agents to the diet and the use of suppositories and enemas may be necessary to achieve regular evacuation. Diarrhoea, if it occurs, may require the use of antidiarrhoeals such as codeine phosphate. Treatment of impotence, if it is due to autonomic neuropathy, is unsatisfactory but may sometimes be relieved by implantation of a mechanical prosthesis into the penis.

Deep vein thrombosis

In acute polyneuritis immobility of the patient may give rise to the problems regularly associated with paralysis and discussed elsewhere (*see* Chapters 7 and 15). A particular hazard may be deep vein thrombosis, so that in addition to prescribing regular active physiotherapy it may be advisable to consider prophylactive anticoagulants such as, for example, subcutaneous heparin 5000 units every 12 h.

Respiratory difficulty

In patients with severe polyneuropathy it is important to monitor carefully the respiratory capacity of the patient, and when this is in doubt regular measurements of peak expiratory flow or vital capacity should be carried out, supplemented if necessary by blood gas analysis. If there is respiratory distress a tracheostomy and management by intermittent positive pressure ventilation in an intensive care unit may be necessary.

REFERENCES

Austin, J H (1958) Recurrent polyneuropathies and their corticosteroid treatment. *Brain*, **81**, 157–192.

Banerji, N K and Hurwitz, L J (1971) Nervous system manifestations after gastric surgery. *Acta Neurologica Scandinavica*, **47**, 485–513.

Bannister, Sir Roger (1979) Chronic autonomic failure with postural hypotension. *Lancet*, **2**, 404–406.

Biemond, A (1970) Femoral neuropathy. In: *Handbook of Clinical Neurology*, vol. 8: *Diseases of Nerves*, pp. 303–310. (Eds) P J Vinken and G W Bruyn. North-Holland Publishing Company, Amsterdam.

Bleehen, S S, Lovelace, R E and Cotton, R E (1963) Mononeuritis multiplex in polyarteritis nodosa. *Quarterly Journal of Medicine*, **32**, 193–209.

Bradley, W G (1974) The neuropathies. In: *Disorders of Voluntary Muscle*, pp. 804–851. (Ed) J N Walton. Churchill Livingstone, Edinburgh.

Brain, Lord, Croft, P B and Wilkinson, M (1969) The carcinomatous neuromyopathies. In: *Recent Advances in Neurology and Neuropsychiatry*, pp. 13–14. (Eds) Lord Brain and M Wilkinson. Churchill Livingstone, London.

Brown, J R and Opitz, J L (1970) Treatment of neuropathies. In: *Handbook of Clinical Neurology*, vol. 8: *Diseases of Nerves*, pp. 373—411. (Eds) P J Vinken and G W Bruyn. North-Holland Publishing Company, Amsterdam.

Bruyn, G W and Garland, H (1970) Neuropathies of endocrine origin. In: *Handbook of Clinical Neurology*, vol. 8: *Diseases of Nerves*, pp. 29—71. (Eds) P J Vinken and G W Bruyn. North-Holland Publishing Company, Amsterdam.

Cooke, W T and Smith, W T (1966) Neurological disorders associated with adult coeliac disease. *Brain*, **89**, 683—722.

Dyck, P J and Lambert, E H (1970) Polyneuropathy associated with hypothyroidism. *Journal of Neuropathology and Experimental Neurology*, **29**, 631—658.

Ekbom, K A (1970) Restless legs. In: *Handbook of Clinical Neurology*, vol. 8: *Diseases of Nerves*, pp. 311—320. (Eds) P J Vinken and G W Bruyn. North-Holland Publishing Company, Amsterdam.

Ferguson, R H and Slocumb, C H (1961) Peripheral neuropathy in rheumatoid arthritis. *Bulletin of Rheumatic Diseases*, **11**, 251—254.

Gargour, G, MacGaffey, K, Locke, S and Stein, M D (1964) Anterior radiculopathy and lupus erythematosus cells. *British Medical Journal*, **2**, 799—801.

Golding, D N (1973) D-penicillamine in rheumatoid arthritis. *British Journal of Hospital Medicine*, **9**, 805—813.

Guillain, G, Barré, J and Strohl, H (1916) Sur un syndrome de radiculonévrite avec hyperalbuminose du liquide cephalorachidien sans réaction cellulaire. *Bulletins et mémoires de la Sociètè medicale des hopitaux de Paris*, **40**, 1462—1470; translated (1968) *Archives of Neurology*, **18**, 450—452.

Gutmann, E and Guttmann, L (1944) Effect of galvanic exercise on denervated and reinnervated muscles in rabbit. *Journal of Neurology, Neurosurgery and Psychiatry*, **7**, 7—17.

Hornstein, O P (1970) Melkersson—Rosenthal syndrome. In: *Handbook of Clinical Neurology*, vol. 8: *Diseases of Nerves*, pp. 205—240. (Eds) P J Vinken and G W Bruyn. North-Holland Publishing Company, Amsterdam.

Hughes, R A C (1978) Acute inflammatory polyneuropathy. *British Journal of Hospital Medicine*, **20**, 688—693.

Hughes, R A C, Newsom-Davis, J M, Perkin, G D and Pierce, J M (1978) Controlled trial of prednisolone in acute polyneuropathy. *Lancet*, **2**, 750—753.

Jackson, R H, Miller, H and Schapira, K (1957) Polyradiculitis (Landry—Guillain—Barré syndrome): treatment with cortisone and corticotrophin. *British Medical Journal*, **1**, 480—484.

Jackson, S (1945) The role of galvanism in the treatment of denervated voluntary muscle in man. *Brain*, **68**, 300—330.

Johnson, R H and Richardson, E P (1968) The neurological manifestations of systemic lupus erythematosus: a clinical—pathological study of 24 cases and review of the literature. *Medicine (Baltimore)*, **47**, 337—369.

Keck, G (1962) The tarsal tunnel syndrome. *Journal of Bone and Joint Surgery*, **44A/1**, 180—182.

Löffel, N B, Rossi, L N, Mumenthaler, M, Lütschg, J and Ludin, H P (1977) The Landry—Guillain—Barré syndrome: complications, prognosis and natural history in 123 cases. *Journal of the Neurological Sciences*, **33**, 71—79.

Matthews, W B (1975) Sarcoid neuropathy. In: *Peripheral Neuropathy*, pp. 1199–1206. (Eds) P J Dyck, P K Thomas and E H Lambert. W B Saunders, Philadelphia.

Mitchell, D M and Olczak, S A (1979) Remission of a syndrome indistinguishable from motor-neurone disease after resection of bronchial carcinoma. *British Medical Journal*, **2**, 176–177.

Murray, I P C and Simpson, J A (1958) Acroparaesthesia in myxoedema; a clinical and electromyographic study. *Lancet*, **2**, 1360–1363.

Osborne, G V (1959) Ulnar neuritis. *Postgraduate Medical Journal*, **35**, 392–396.

Parsonage, M J and Turner, J W A (1948) Neuralgic amyotrophy: the shoulder girdle syndrome. *Lancet*, **1**, 973–978.

Raff, M C, Sangalang, V and Asbury, A K (1968) Ischaemic mononeuropathy multiplex associated with diabetes mellitus. *Archives of Neurology (Chicago)*, **18**, 487–499.

Ridley, A (1969) The neuropathy of acute intermittent porphyria. *Quarterly Journal of Medicine*, **38**, 307–333.

Riley, C M, Day, R L, Greeley, D McL and Langford, W S (1949) Central autonomic dysfunction with defective lachrymation, 1. Report of five cases. *Pediatrics*, **3**, 468–478.

Rosen, A D and Vastola, E F (1976) Clinical effects of cyclophosphamide in Guillain–Barré polyneuritis. *Journal of the Neurological Sciences*, **30**, 179–187.

Seddon, H J (1943) Three types of nerve injury. *Brain*, **66**, 237–288.

Seddon, Sir Herbert (1975) *Surgical disorders of the peripheral nerves*, 2nd edn. Churchill Livingstone, Edinburgh.

Shy, G M and Drager, G A (1960) A neurological syndrome associated with orthostatic hypotension. *Archives of Neurology (Chicago)*, **2**, 511–527.

Sidey, J D (1969) Weak ankles. A study of common peroneal nerve entrapment neuropathy. *British Medical Journal*, **3**, 623–626.

Steinberg, D, Mize, C E, Herndon, J H Jr, Fales, H M, Engel, W K and Vroom, F Q (1970) Phytanic acid in patients with Refsum's syndrome and response to dietary treatment. *Archives of Internal Medicine*, **125**, 75–87.

Stevens, H (1957) Meralgia paraesthetica. *Archives of Neurology and Psychiatry*, **77**, 557–574.

Sunderland, S (1978) *Nerves and nerve injuries*, 2nd edn. Churchill Livingstone, Edinburgh and London.

Taverner, D (1959) The prognosis and treatment of spontaneous facial palsy. *Proceedings of the Royal Society of Medicine*, **52**, 1077–1080.

Taverner, D, Cohen, S B and Hutchinson, B C (1971) Comparison of corticotrophin and prednisolone in treatment of idiopathic facial paralysis (Bell's palsy). *British Medical Journal*, **4**, 20–22.

Thomas, P K and Lascelles, R G (1965) Schwann cell abnormalities in diabetic neuropathy. *Lancet*, **1**, 1355–1357.

Thomas, P K, Lascelles, R G, Hallpike, J F and Hewer, R L (1969) Recurrent and chronic relapsing Guillain–Barré polyneuritis. *Brain*, **92**, 589–606.

Yuill, G M, Swinburn, W R and Liversedge, L A (1970) Treatment of polyneuropathy with azathioprine. *Lancet*, **2**, 854–856.

CHAPTER THIRTEEN

Myasthenia Gravis and Myasthenic Syndrome

PATHOPHYSIOLOGY

The earliest evidence for a defect of neuromuscular transmission in myasthenia gravis was provided by Jolly in 1895 when he showed that a faradic stimulus to a muscle in an affected patient was followed by a brisk contraction and then a falling off in tension. It was not, however, until 1934 when Mary Walker demonstrated the value of physostigmine in treatment that the defect was clearly shown to be one of neuro-muscular transmission. Later studies, which have shown that repetitive stimulation of a peripheral nerve in myasthenia gravis is accompanied by a progressive fall in the amplitude of action potentials evoked in the muscles supplied by the nerve, have confirmed the nature of the defect. Until quite recently, however, it has not been certain whether the site of the disturbance in neuromuscular transmission is pre-junctional, that is due to a failure of production or release of acetylcholine from the nerve ending, or post-junctional due to interference with its action at the motor end-plate. A crucial experiment was that of Elmqvist *et al.* (1964) who showed that in excised intercostal muscle from patients with myasthenia gravis miniature end-plate potentials occur at normal frequency with an amplitude reduced to about one-fifth of normal. This was taken to mean that the defect in myasthenia gravis was likely to be pre-junctional and could be explained in terms of a reduced quantity of acetylcholine in the transmitter particles which pass from the nerve endings to the muscle membrane. Subsequent work, however, has shown that the motor end-plate in myasthenic muscle is less sensitive to acetylcholine applied by micro-iontophoretic injection (Albuquerque *et al.*, 1976) and it has also been shown that the number of acetylcho-line receptors in myasthenic muscle is reduced (Fambrough *et al.*, 1973).

It is now evident that in myasthenia gravis the fundamental defect is in the immune system and that the defect in neuromuscular conduction is caused by antibodies to acetylcholine receptor. In 1960 Simpson drew attention to the frequent association between myasthenia gravis and other disorders considered to be autoimmune, such as rheumatoid arthritis and thyroid disease. The occurrence of neonatal myasthenia in a proportion of children of myasthenic mothers could be explained by an abnormal reaction of the infant's muscle to maternal antibody transmitted through the placenta. The presence of abnormalities in the thymus of patients with myasthenia gravis, and the association with thymic tumour, is also significant in relation to the now clearly recognised role of the thymus in immune function. Further evidence for an immunological relationship came from the observation that many patients with myasthenia have antibodies which bind to the striations of skeletal muscle (Strauss *et al.*, 1966). In 1973 Patrick and Lindstrom produced a myasthenic syndrome in rabbits by injecting acetylcholine receptor prepared from the electric eel and mixed with adjuvant, and experimental autoimmune myasthenia gravis has since been induced in a variety of animal species. The development of experimental autoimmune myasthenia gravis can be blocked by neonatal thymectomy or by treatment either with hydrocortisone or azathioprine (Abramsky *et al.*, 1976). Antibodies to human acetylcholine receptor have been found in patients with myasthenia gravis (Lindstrom *et al.*, 1976) and in infants with neonatal myasthenia, antibodies similar to those present in the mother have been found (Keesey *et al.*, 1977).

It is of interest that in common with other diseases where there is abnormality in the immune response there has been found to be a strong association between myasthenia gravis and a particular HLA antigen, namely HLA 8 (Behan *et al.*, 1973).

PROGNOSIS

Myasthenia gravis may occur at any age, but most commonly between 20 and 30 when there is a marked preponderance of females to males. In the early stages the course is difficult to predict; some cases progressing steadily, others going into remission or remaining static. If the condition remains confined to the extra-ocular muscles the prognosis for life expectancy and disability is excellent. On the other hand patients who have a thymic tumour, which is found in 10—20 per cent of cases, have a much less favourable outlook. In general the mortality is greatest during the first year, and from 4 to 7 years after the onset, deaths rarely occurring later than 10 years from the onset of the illness (Simpson, 1958).

ANTICHOLINESTERASE DRUGS

For many years these drugs have been the mainstay of the treatment of myasthenia gravis. In addition to providing maintenance therapy, which in many instances will control the symptoms of myasthenia, they are also useful in confirming the diagnosis since a test dose in an affected patient will generally produce temporary relief of symptoms. The following are the most generally useful drugs.

Edrophonium chloride (Tensilon)

This drug, which may be given i.m. or i.v., has a short duration of action which makes it ineffective as a form of treatment but extremely valuable when used as a diagnostic test. Its particular value in treatment lies in the fact that a Tensilon test may make it possible to distinguish deterioration in a patient's condition due to a myasthenic crisis from that due to cholinergic block. When used for a diagnostic test 10 mg in 1 ml of solution is given i.v. Initially a test dose of 2 mg is given to ascertain if the patient is sensitive and if the patient does not react the rest of the dose is given after an interval of ½ min. If the weakness is due to myasthenia improvement occurs after about 1 min and persists for up to about 5 min. A healthy subject may experience a tight sensation round the eyes and fasciculation may be seen in this area for a few seconds. In a cholinergic crisis these features may be increased, weakness may become more pronounced, and there is a risk that respiratory weakness may occur. When the drug is given in a suspected cholinergic crisis it is therefore advisable to precede its administration by an injection of 0.3–0.6 mg of atropine sulphate and it is important that facilities for resuscitation, including assisted respiration, should be available.

Neostigmine bromide (Prostigmin)

This drug is an anticholinesterase which is made up in 15 mg tablets and which has a duration of action of 2–6 h. In mild cases it may be given in as low a dose as half a tablet three times a day, but a few patients may require as many as 30 tablets in the day given in divided doses of three tablets every 2 h. The most suitable time of administration is ½ h before a meal, particularly if the patient has difficulty in chewing or swallowing. Neostigmine methyl sulphate is suitable for injection and 1 mg is equivalent to one 15 mg tablet of neostigmine bromide. It may be given by s.c. or i.m. injection but should not be used intravenously as there is a risk of cardiac arrest. When neostigmine is given by injection it should be preceded by atropine sulphate (0.5 mg). Neostigmine methyl sulphate by injection can be used as a diagnostic test for myasthenia gravis but its longer duration of action makes it a less satisfactory test than Tensilon and for this reason it is not satisfactory as a test for distinguishing between a myasthenic and a cholinergic crisis. In severe cases of myasthenia it may be necessary to give neostigmine by injection and this is the route of administration which should be employed when treating a myasthenic crisis. Occasionally neostigmine tablets may give rise to cholinergic side-effects such as colic and sweating, and if this is the case atropine sulphate 0.6 mg orally or propantheline bromide (15 mg) may be given, but this is undesirable and is best avoided, as it may mask physical signs such as constriction of the pupil which may indicate the development of a cholinergic crisis.

Pyridostigmine bromide (Mestinon)

Pyridostigmine is made up in 60 mg tablets each of which is equivalent to one 15 mg tablet of neostigmine bromide. The duration of action is slightly more prolonged than that of neostigmine and because the effect builds up and declines more slowly it gives smoother control of effect than neostigmine and many patients find it preferable. It also has a weaker muscarinic action than neostigmine and is therefore less likely to give rise to cholinergic side-effects. It is also made up in ampoules containing 1 mg of pyridostigmine bromide which can be given by s.c. or i.m. injection.

Ambenonium chloride (Mytelase)

This is a cholinergic drug which is made up in tablets of 10 mg of ambenonium chloride; 25 mg is approximately equivalent to 15 mg of neostigmine bromide. Its duration of action is slightly longer than pyridostigmine but although muscarinic side-effects are less common than with either pyridostigmine or neostigmine it carries a greater risk of giving rise to a cholinergic crisis. For this reason it is advisable always to start with a small dose (5 mg) and to build up the dose very gradually according to the needs of the patient. It should not be given along with other antimyasthenic drugs. It may occasionally be indicated if the patient is sensitive to bromide.

Of the cholinergic drugs pyridostigmine is probably the most generally acceptable to patients and is the most suitable drug for maintenance therapy. Because of its more abrupt onset of effect neostigmine is more suitable for treatment when myasthenia is in an acute phase. Ephedrine sulphate in a dose of 25 mg three times a day by mouth (Edgeworth, 1930) is sometimes used as an adjuvant to cholinergic drugs but it is of doubtful value and its mode of action is uncertain. Potassium chloride can also be given to potentiate the action of cholinergic drugs or alternatively spironolactone (400 mg per day) can be given to conserve potassium but the value of either of these measures is marginal.

THYMECTOMY

Many studies have been carried out on the effects of thymectomy on myasthenia gravis since Blalock introduced the operation in 1936. There is general agreement that the majority of patients with myasthenia gravis who undergo thymectomy can expect a substantial degree of improvement, and that the outlook for patients who have the operation is considerably better than in those who are treated conservatively. This applies particularly to patients who do not have a thymoma, but even in those who have a tumour a proportion can expect to benefit (Simpson, 1958; Perlo *et al.*, 1966; Buckingham *et al.*, 1976). Nevertheless it remains difficult to predict the outcome of surgery in an individual patient and the indications for operation remain imprecise. Certain guidelines, however, have become evident. Thus the strongest prospect for remission appears to be with young patients who have had the disease for a relatively short time. Since the mortality from myasthenia gravis is greatest in the first 5 years after the onset of the disease there is a significant risk to life during this period in patients who are treated conservatively. The most definite indication for surgery is therefore in young patients who have had the disease for a relatively short time and in whom the condition is severe or generalised. This applies particularly to young women who tend on the whole to respond more favourably to thymectomy than males. On the other hand, patients in whom the myasthenic symptoms have been confined and remain confined to the extra-ocular muscles have such an excellent prognosis, in respect both of life and the disease becoming progressive, that it would appear that surgery has little to offer. With the older patient who has had the disease for more than 5 years the decision is more difficult. Here a balance has to be reached between the degree of disability and its tendency to progress, on the one hand, and the possible hazards and benefits of surgery on the other; taking into account that at this stage the mortality from conservatively treated myasthenia should be very small. If a thymoma is present the outlook is less favourable whether or not surgery is carried out, but it does appear that, in this situation also, patients do better if the thymus is removed. Moreover, although patients with thymomas are more likely to die of the effects of the myasthenia than of the tumour these tumours are frequently locally invasive. It has been held that the outlook is improved if the patient has radiotherapy before operation (Keynes, 1954; Perlo *et al.*, 1966) but this view is not firmly established (Simpson, 1974).

The main hazard of thymectomy lies in the unpredictable nature of the response of the patient to the operation. Frequently there is a rapid but temporary improvement during the immediate post-operative period when no neostigmine may be necessary, and then after the third or fourth day there may be a progressive increase in the need for medication which may be followed by a gradual improvement. This improvement may take place very gradually so that the maximum benefit may not be seen until the third post-operative year. During the early days after operation when an initial improvement takes place it is important to guard against the development of a cholinergic crisis which may readily develop if too much neostigmine is given. The patient should be nursed in an intensive care situation with facilities for positive pressure respiration and tracheostomy, if necessary, and during the early days after the operation it is best to use neostigmine in preference to pyridostigmine, and to administer it subcutaneously.

The traditional surgical technique for thymectomy is one in which the sternum is split. This is a relatively major procedure which in the past has carried a significant mortality although this is now much reduced. A less formidable operation is that of transcervical thymectomy in which the thymus is extracted from the mediastinum using mediastinoscopy (Kirschner *et al.*, 1969; Genkins *et al.*, 1975). This operation has the advantage that it can be considered for patients for whom the possible risks of transcervical thymectomy would not seem to be justified. On the other hand with this procedure it is less easy to be certain that the whole thymus has been removed.

STEROIDS AND OTHER IMMUNOSUPPRESSIVE DRUGS

When treatment with ACTH was first introduced on an empirical basis it was found that although some patients improved there might be a period of deterioration before this took place (Torda and Wolff, 1949). Since that time many studies of steroid therapy have been carried out and although these are in the main uncontrolled they have generally shown that the seriously ill patient with myasthenia gravis can be expected to improve, either with parenteral ACTH, with prednisone by mouth, or with other immunosuppressive drugs such as azathioprine (Rowland, 1978). Steroids are probably not indicated in mildly affected patients who can be managed adequately on pyridostigmine, or in patients for whom there is a clear indication for thymectomy, but may be appropriate for seriously ill patients who are not suitable for thymectomy or who have had the operation and remain ill in spite of the procedure. They may also be indicated in patients whose disease is of long standing and who have developed atrophic changes in the affected muscles which have become resistant to neostigmine. In view of the possibility of initial deterioration after starting treatment it is advisable to commence therapy with steroids in hospital and to start with a small dose (for example, prednisolone 25 mg on alternate days) which is gradually increased. With prednisolone a recommended maintenance dose is 50 mg daily or 100 mg on alternate days. This dose may be continued for several months and then gradually reduced (Patten, 1978). The indications for other immunosuppressive drugs (Rowland, 1971) are not firmly established but these should probably be reserved for patients who do not respond adequately to steroids. Other measures which may prove helpful in refractory cases include i.m. injections of 10–20 ml of human γ-globulin every 3 weeks, thoracic duct drainage and plasma exchange. With thoracic duct drainage the response may be rapid but is short-lived. Plasma exchange may also achieve rapid improvement which, when the treatment is combined with immunosuppressive drugs, can be maintained for long periods. Its application, however, requires considerable resources, and possible complications include reactions to foreign substances, infection and haemorrhage (Behan *et al.*, 1979).

MYASTHENIC CRISIS

A myasthenic crisis may occur at any time in the course of the patient's illness but may be brought on characteristically by intercurrent infection, fatigue, too warm an environment or even emotional disturbance. Drugs which may cause neuromuscular block include chlorpromazine, ether, quinidine and quinine; because of the effect of the latter drug patients should avoid tonic water. Antibiotics such as streptomycin, neomycin, gentamycin, polymyxin and colistin may cause a neuromuscular block which can be partially reversed by calcium. The administration of an enema has been known to precipitate a myasthenic crisis, possibly by causing potassium depletion.

If a patient with myasthenia has a sudden exacerbation of weakness it is important to administer a test dose of Tensilon to establish the presence of a myasthenic block and then to control the myasthenic state with i.m. injections of neostigmine. It is important that the patient should be nursed in a situation where facilities for intensive care are available so that intubation and positive pressure ventilation can be initiated if there is respiratory failure or bulbar paralysis.

CHOLINERGIC PARALYSIS

If a patient who is receiving treatment with neostigmine or pyridostigmine develops muscarinic side-effects such as colic, sweating, salivation and constriction of the pupil, these signs may indicate a cholinergic crisis is impending. It is therefore undesirable to block muscarinic side-effects with atropine in a patient who is receiving maintenance therapy for myasthenia. If weakness develops in this situation it is necessary to confirm the diagnosis of cholinergic crisis by means of an edrophonium test. If edrophonium is given in this situation it is essential that an injection of atropine should be given first and that facilities should be available for assisted respiration. The treatment of paralysis due to a cholinergic crisis depends essentially on maintaining respiration, while at the same time atropine sulphate (2 mg) is injected intravenously 2-hourly until toxic signs appear. Once clinical improvement has set in, the patient's condition should be assessed by the edrophonium test and when a myasthenic type of response has occurred treatment with neostigmine may be cautiously resumed, administering the drug initially by i.m. injection.

EATON—LAMBERT SYNDROME

In 1957 Eaton and Lambert reported on the electrophysiological findings in patients with a myasthenia-like syndrome occurring in association with carcinoma. The association between bronchial carcinoma and the myasthenia-like syndrome had previously been recognised by Anderson *et al.* (1953). In this condition there may be proximal weakness and fatiguability associated with diminished or absent tendon reflexes, but with little consistent response to neostigmine or Tensilon. Repetitive stimulation of a peripheral nerve evokes smaller than normal action potentials in the muscle supplied, which increase in amplitude with tetanisation. Microelectrode studies of excised intercostal muscle have shown normal miniature end-plate potentials but with an abnormal end-plate response during nerve stimulation consistent with a pre-junctional block similar to the defect which would arise from too much magnesium or exposure to botulinus toxin (Lambert and Elmqvist, 1971). Agents which promote the release of acetylcholine from the nerve ending may be beneficial, and the most widely used has been guanidine hydrochloride in a dose of 25—50 mg/kg body-weight daily in divided doses, but this carries a risk of bone marrow depression.

REFERENCES

Abramsky, O, Tarrab-Hazdai, R, Aharonov, A and Fuchs, S (1976) Immunosuppression of experimental autoimmune myasthenia gravis by hydrocortisone and azathioprine. *Journal of Immunology*, **117**, 225—228.

Albuquerque, E X, Rash, J E, Mayer, R F and Satterfield, J R (1976) An electrophysiological and morphological study of the neuromuscular junction in patients with myasthenia gravis. *Experimental Neurology*, **51**, 536—563.

Anderson, H J, Churchill-Davidson, H C and Richardson, A T (1953) Bronchial neoplasm with myasthenia. Prolonged apnoea after administration of succinylcholine. *Lancet*, **2**, 1291—1293.

Behan, P O, Simpson, J A and Dyck, H (1973) Immune response genes in myasthenia gravis. *Lancet*, **2**, 1033.

Behan, P O, Shakir, R A, Simpson, J A, Burnett, A K, Allan, T L and Haase, G (1979) Plasma-exchange combined with immunosuppressive therapy in myasthenia gravis. *Lancet*, **2**, 438—440.

Buckingham, J M, Howard, F M Jr, Bernatz, P E, Payne, W S, Harrison, E G Jr, O'Brien, P C and Weiland, L N (1976) The value of thymectomy in myasthenia gravis. A computer adjusted matched study. *Annals of Surgery*, **184**, 453—458.

Eaton, L M and Lambert, E H (1956) Electromyography and electric stimulation of nerves in diseases of motor unit. Observations on myasthenic syndrome associated with malignant tumours. *Journal of the American Medical Association*, **163**, 1117—1124.

Edgeworth, H (1930) A report of progress and the use of ephedrine in a case of myasthenia gravis. *Journal of the American Medical Association*, **94**, 1136.

Elmqvist, D, Hofmann, W W, Kugelberg, E and Quastel, D M J (1964) An electrophysiological investigation of neuromuscular transmission in myasthenia gravis. *Journal of Physiology*, **174**, 417—434.

Fambrough, D M, Drachman, D B and Satyamurti, S (1973) Neuromuscular junction in myasthenia gravis: decreased acetylcholine receptors. *Science*, **182**, 293—295.

Genkins, G, Papatestas, A E, Horowitz, S H and Kornfield, P (1975) Studies on myasthenia gravis: early thymectomy. Electrophysiologic and pathologic correlations. *American Journal of Medicine*, **58**, 517—524.

Jolly, F (1895) Über myasthenia gravis pseudoparalytica. *Berliner Klinische Wochenschrift*, **32**, 33—34.

Keesey, J, Lindstrom, J, Cokely, H and Hermann, C Jr (1977) Anti-acetylcholine receptor antibody in neonatal myasthenia gravis. *New England Journal of Medicine*, **296**, 55.

Keynes, G (1954) Surgery of the thymus gland. Second (and third) thoughts. *Lancet*, **1**, 1197—1202.

Kirschner, P A, Osserman, K E and Kark, A E (1969) Studies in myasthenia gravis. Transcervical total thymectomy. *Journal of the American Medical Association*, **209**, 906–910.

Lambert, E H and Elmqvist, D (1971) Quantal components of end-plate potentials in the myasthenic syndrome. *Annals of the New York Academy of Sciences*, **183**, 183–199.

Lindstrom, J M, Seybold, M E, Lennon, V A and Lambert, E H (1976) Antibody to acetylcholine receptor in myasthenia gravis. Prevalence, clinical correlates, and diagnostic value. *Neurology (Minneapolis)*, **26**, 1054–1059.

Patrick, J and Lindstrom, J (1973) Autoimmune response to acetylcholine receptor. *Science*, **180**, 871–872.

Patten, B M (1978) Myasthenia gravis: review of diagnosis and management. *Muscle and Nerve*, **1**, 190–205.

Perlo, V P, Poskanzer, D C, Schwab, R S, Viets, H R, Osserman, K E and Genkins, G (1966) Myasthenia gravis: evaluation of treatment in 1335 patients. *Neurology (Minneapolis)*, **16**, 431–439.

Rowland, L P (1971) Immunosuppressive drugs for the treatment of myasthenia gravis. *Annals of the New York Academy of Sciences*, **183**, 351–357.

Rowland, L P (1978) Myasthenia gravis. In: *Recent Advances in Clinical Neurology*, No. 2. (Eds) W B Matthews and G H Glaser. Churchill Livingstone, Edinburgh and London.

Simpson, J A (1958) An evaluation of thymectomy in myasthenia gravis. *Brain*, **81**, 112–144.

Simpson, J A (1960) Myasthenia gravis: a new hypothesis. *Scottish Medical Journal*, **5**, 419–436.

Simpson, J A (1974) Myasthenia gravis and myasthenic syndromes. In: *Disorders of Voluntary Muscle*, 3rd edn. (Ed) J N Walton. Churchill Livingstone, Edinburgh and London.

Strauss, A J J, Smith, C W, Case, G W, Van der Geld, H W R, McFarlin, D E and Barlow, M (1966) Further studies on the specificity of the presumed immune associations of myasthenia gravis. *Annals of the New York Academy of Sciences*, **135**, 557–579.

Torda, C and Wolff, H G (1949) Effects of adrenocorticotrophic hormone on neuromuscular junction in patients with myasthenia gravis. *Journal of Clinical Investigation*, **28**, 1228–1235.

Walker, M B (1934) Treatment of myasthenia gravis with prostigmine. *Lancet*, **1**, 1200–1201.

CHAPTER FOURTEEN

Disorders of Muscle

Disorders of voluntary muscle include a number of acquired diseases such as polymyositis, a number of myopathies, some of which are acquired and some of which have a genetic basis, which are associated with endocrine or metabolic disorders, and a large group of inherited diseases which include the muscular dystrophies and the congenital myopathies. In the acquired myopathies and those associated with metabolic disturbance treatment is frequently available and is dependent on a clear understanding of the nature of the underlying disorder. In many of the genetically determined disorders of muscle there is no definitive treatment but careful management of particular problems may contribute to the welfare of the patient. In many of these disorders a major problem is one of appropriate genetic counselling and this depends both on accurate diagnosis and on as full as possible a knowledge of the mode of transmission of the particular disorder.

POLYMYOSITIS

Pathophysiology and prognosis

This disorder, which can occur at any time of life from infancy to old age, has been classified by the World Federation of Neurology Research Group on Neuromuscular Disorders (1968) into three varieties:

(1) type alpha: uncomplicated polymyositis;
(2) type beta: dermatomyositis and myositis in association with connective tissue disorders;
(3) type gamma: polymyositis associated with malignancy.

Typically the pathological changes in the muscle comprise degenerative changes in the muscle fibres together with evidence of regeneration and infiltration of inflammatory cells. The degree of infiltration is very variable and if it is not marked it may be difficult to distinguish the condition pathologically from limb-girdle muscular dystrophy. The association of the disease with connective tissue disorders such as systemic lupus erythematosus, and the clinical improvement in the condition which may result from the immunosuppressive therapy, suggest that the condition may have an immunological basis. Moreover many patients with the disease have high levels of serum globulin and Dawkins (1965) has induced experimental myositis in animals by injection of muscle tissue together with adjuvant. The association of polymyositis with malignancy could also be explained on an immune basis and there are a number of reports of virus particles in specimens of muscle from patients with polymyositis (Chou and Gutmann, 1970; Mastaglia and Walton, 1971) which could be consistent with the possibility that in some cases the disease may be due to hypersensitivity to a virus agent. Cases of dermatomyositis have sometimes been associated with high antibody titres to Coxsackie B viruses (Dubowitz, 1978). This group of viruses is also associated with Bornholm disease, in which there is acute tenderness of the intercostal muscles. The prognosis and natural history of polymyositis are very variable. Sometimes the disease runs a self-limiting course with spontaneous recovery but in other patients it runs a relatively chronic course and the patient is left with some permanent weakness of the muscles. With other patients, and this is particularly so when the condition is associated with malignancies, it may run a progressive course with a fatal outcome. Sometimes it runs an acute course with rapid progression to involve the respiratory and bulbar muscles.

Steroids — immunosuppression

Sometimes the condition in its presentation is very similar to limb-girdle muscular dystrophy and it is important to establish a precise diagnosis wherever possible to exclude a genetically determined disorder. Careful clinical assessment is therefore important together with full investigation including muscle biopsy and electromyography. The general management of the patient is particularly important as the patient must be rested in the acute stage but at the same time active movement of the limbs should be encouraged to prevent the development of contractures. If the disease is severe and progressive, involvement of the respiratory and bulbar muscles may necessitate positive pressure respiration. The majority of patients will respond favourably to treatment with steroids and the response to treatment may be judged both by an increase in strength in the patients and a decline in the serum enzyme levels for creatine phosphokinase and aldolase. In acute or subacute cases improvement may be followed by a gradual return to completely normal function. In the chronic cases improvement may be less marked and the patient is frequently left with residual weakness. It is generally recommended that treatment should be started with a high dose of prednisolone such as for an adult 60 mg daily in divided doses. As the patient improves the dosage may be lowered and then maintenance therapy with a dose of between 7.5 and 20 mg daily may be continued. Sometimes after 6 months to a year it may be possible to discontinue therapy altogether, but some patients require maintenance therapy for several years or longer. With long-term therapy great care must be exercised in avoiding potassium depletion and it may be necessary to administer antacids by mouth. Some patients respond poorly to steroids and, if this is the case, the treatment may be supplemented by immunosuppressive drugs such as azathioprine 100 mg once or twice daily. Alternatively cyclophosphamide may be given in a starting dose of 50 mg twice daily increasing to 300 mg daily, monitoring the treatment with serum creatine kinase levels and with red and white cell blood counts (Pearson and Currie, 1974).

Dubowitz (1978) has commented on the possible hazards of overtreatment with steroids which may give rise to a steroid myopathy in place of the original myositis. He recommends the administration of prednisolone in moderate dosage and for a limited period of time, and suggests a dose of 1 mg/kg body-weight daily until the response to treatment is evident; gradually reducing the dosage with a view to discontinuing altogether within about 6 months. He also suggests that the importance of a declining level of serum enzymes as a monitor of therapy has been over-emphasised and that the clinical return of muscle power is the most important guide.

POLYMYALGIA RHEUMATICA

This is a condition of the middle-aged or elderly in which the problem is one of pain and stiffness in the muscles, usually of the shoulder girdle and sometimes of the pelvic girdle, most marked in the morning. Muscular weakness is generally not a feature. It is associated with a high erythrocyte sedimentation rate and is particularly likely to be associated with cranial or temporal arteritis. Over the long term it is a self-limiting condition generally resolving in about 3 years, and if it is associated with cranial arteritis there is a risk that visual failure or blindness may develop. It responds rapidly to treatment with corticosteroids and prednisolone may be given in a dose of 10–15 mg daily. If cranial arteritis is also present a much higher dose of 60–100 mg should be given promptly in view of the danger of visual failure developing. This may be reduced to a maintenance dose as the symptoms resolve and the ESR falls to normal.

METABOLIC MYOPATHY

Periodic paralysis

This group of disorders is characterised by dominant inheritance and episodes of flaccid paralysis in which the plasma potassium may fall or be elevated, or in the normokalaemic form remain normal.

Hypokalaemic periodic paralysis

In this condition attacks of severe weakness occur, particularly in the early morning on wakening, and may last from a few hours to a few days. These attacks are particularly liable to occur following a period of rest after vigorous exercise or following a large carbohydrate meal, and a clinical attack may be induced by taking glucose accompanied by insulin. The plasma potassium falls during an attack and returns to normal during recovery. An acute attack may be treated by giving potassium chloride up to about 10 g by mouth and this can be repeated after 2 h. In severe paralysis it may be necessary to give the potassium intravenously. The use of potassium chloride prophylactically is of limited value but slowly released potassium in the form of slow-K, taken together with a low carbohydrate diet, may be helpful. Griggs *et al.* (1970) found that acetazolamide in a dose of 125—250 mg twice or three times a day was effective, and McArdle (1974) has used chlorothiazide 250 mg daily or the carbonic anhydrase inhibitor dichlorphenamide (Daranide) 50 mg daily along with slow-K. In general the long-term prognosis is favourable as attacks tend to diminish as the patient becomes older.

Thyrotoxic periodic paralysis

A form of periodic paralysis may occur in association with thyrotoxicosis. It is similar in its clinical features to hypokalaemic periodic paralysis but responds to treatment of the thyrotoxicosis. This condition occurs most frequently in Chinese or Japanese males and a family history is unusual.

Hyperkalaemic periodic paralysis

Unlike hypokalaemic periodic paralysis, which occurs particularly in adults, this condition is more likely to occur in childhood. Exercise is an important predisposing factor and an attack is particularly liable to occur when resting in a chair perhaps ½ h after exercise. Other factors are cold, or missing a meal. Attacks are relatively brief and last from ½ h to 2–3 h and they are accompanied by elevation of the plasma potassium which may rise to levels of up to 7 mmol/l. An attack when it occurs is seldom severe enough to require treatment, and if treatment is necessary intravenous calcium gluconate in a dose of 1–2 g can be effective. If this does not bring relief then chlorothiazide intravenously or glucose and insulin may be helpful. Acetazolamide or dichlorphenamide are both effective as prophylaxis but chlorothiazide in a dose of about 500 mg per day appears to be the most satisfactory treatment at present.

Normokalaemic periodic paralysis

This condition clinically resembles hyperkalaemic periodic paralysis but the attacks are all severe and persistent and tend to occur at night, lasting sometimes for several days at a time. The paralysis is not accompanied by changes in the blood potassium and in an acute attack may be relieved by a large dose of sodium chloride. A family described by Poskanzer and Kerr (1961) was effectively protected from attacks by taking a combination of 250 mg acetazolamide and 0.1 mg of 9 α-fluorohydrocortisone daily. A family described by Meyers *et al.* (1972) was not helped by acetazolamide.

THE GLYCOGEN STORAGE DISORDERS

The glycogen storage disorders which affect muscle include:

(1) type II α-1,4 glucosidase deficiency (acid maltase) deficiency — Pompe's disease;
(2) type III amylo-1,6 glucosidase (debranching enzyme) deficiency — Forbes' or Cori's disease;
(3) type V myophosphorylase deficiency — McArdle's disease;
(4) type VII phosphofructokinase deficiency — Tarui's disease.

Pompe's disease or acid maltase deficiency is generally fatal in infancy but a milder form exists which may resemble limb-girdle muscular dystrophy. The mild form runs a relatively benign course and no treatment has been effective for the severe form. In Cori's disease muscular weakness and hypotonia is relatively mild and the main problems arise from hepatomegaly so that a high protein intake with frequent small feeds may be advisable to prevent hypoglycaemia (Fernandez and van de Kamer, 1968). In McArdle's disease or myophosphorylase deficiency the clinical picture includes muscle cramps, fatigue, myoglobinuria and weakness, and stiffness during slight or moderate exercise. In management it is important to avoid severe exercise which may bring on the muscle cramps; although taking glucose or fructose may increase exercise tolerance this is of little value as a long-term measure. There is some evidence that exercise tolerance may be increased by a diet rich in fats (Viskoper *et al.*, 1975). Drugs which increase the free fatty acids in plasma such as isoprenaline 10–20 mg, its slow release form Saventrine 30 mg or fenfluramine (Ponderax) 20 mg twice daily have also been tried but are not always tolerated (McArdle, 1974).

ENDOCRINE MYOPATHY

Thyrotoxicosis is frequently associated with a proximal myopathy. Although severe weakness is not very common electromyographic abnormalities have been found in many patients with hyperthyroidism (Ramsay, 1966). This condition generally recovers with adequate treatment of the thyrotoxicosis. Cushing's syndrome may also be associated with muscular weakness particularly of the pelvic girdle. The response to treatment in this condition, however, is less favourable than with thyrotoxic myopathy (Müller and Kugelberg, 1959). Treatment with corticosteroids may also give rise to muscular weakness (Perkoff *et al.*, 1959). This myopathy is particularly likely to develop with steroids which have a fluorine atom in the 9α position, such as triamcinalone. This myopathy is associated with selective atrophy of type II fibres and it tends to resolve if steroid therapy is withdrawn. A painful proximal myopathy may also occur in association with hyperparathyroidism or with osteomalacia and is again associated with atrophy of type II muscle fibres. In hyperparathyroidism the myopathy may resolve if the adenoma is removed. In osteomalacia the myopathy generally responds to administration of vitamin D.

MALIGNANT HYPERPYREXIA

In this condition, which is inherited as an autosomal dominant, the patient is well except when exposed to general anaesthesia although some susceptible subjects have a mild degree of weakness and an elevated serum creatine kinase. During anaesthesia the patient develops a metabolic acidosis in association with tachycardia, rigidity and hyperpyrexia and the condition is frequently fatal. During an attack the serum creatine kinase is markedly elevated and there is also an elevated serum potassium. It is brought about particularly by anaesthetics and muscle-relaxants such as halothane and succinylcholine. The underlying abnormality is thought to be an impairment of the binding of calcium ions to the membrane of the sarcoplasmic reticulum. Unfortunately, not all susceptible subjects have an elevated serum creatine kinase and to establish the diagnosis a muscle biopsy specimen is exposed to a provocative agent such as halothane. The contracture which results may be partially blocked by procaine (Moulds and Denborough, 1972 and 1974).

The possibility of susceptibility must be considered in any patient with a family history of severe reaction to anaesthesia. If general anaesthesia is essential, thiopentone or nitrous oxide with tubocurarine as a relaxant are probably the least hazardous agents but it is doubtful if any general anaesthetic is completely free of risk and spinal or local anaesthesia should be used if possible. If hyperpyrexia develops it is treated by discontinuing the anaesthetic, cooling the patient and correcting the acidosis with intravenous sodium bicarbonate. Intravenous procaine (1 per cent i.v. with a loading dose of 30—40 mg/kg followed by an infusion of 0.2 mg/kg per minute) or procainamide may be helpful but carries a risk of hypotension and its administration should be monitored by the electrocardiogram. Mannitol may be given (1 g/kg i.v.) and steroids in high dosage, either as dexamethasone or i.v. hydrocortisone have given encouraging results. Dantrolene is effective in inhibiting halothane-induced contracture and may be given intravenously in a dose of 1 mg/kg. This may be followed by infusion up to a maximum total dose of 10 mg/kg (Relton *et al.*, 1972; Isaacs and Barlow, 1973; Ellis *et al.*, 1974; Ellis and Halsall, 1980).

MUSCULAR DYSTROPHY

The term muscular dystrophy has been applied to a variety of genetically determined disorders of voluntary muscle which differ widely in their clinical features and mode of presentation. Their classification is difficult but important because management depends on understanding the mode of inheritance, natural history and prognosis, and this depends on precise diagnosis. The muscular dystrophies can be subdivided into major groups which include the 'pure' muscular dystrophies, the myotonias and the congenital myopathies. The following classification of the 'pure' muscular dystrophies is derived from Walton and Gardner-Medwin (1974):

(a) X-linked muscular dystrophy — severe (Duchenne type), benign (Becker type);
(b) autosomal recessive muscular dystrophy — limb-girdle types, childhood muscular dystrophy (except Duchenne), congenital muscular dystrophies;
(c) facioscapulohumeral muscular dystrophy;
(d) distal muscular dystrophy;
(e) ocular muscular dystrophy;
(f) oculopharyngeal muscular dystrophy.

Duchenne muscular dystrophy

In this common form of muscular dystrophy progress is relatively rapid and it is unusual for the child to remain ambulant beyond the age of 12 years or survive beyond the age of 20. There is at present no means of halting the progress of the disease but appropriate care and management can significantly affect the quality of life. Once the child is confined to a wheelchair it is difficult to prevent the development of contractures and deformities, and it is important that he should remain ambulant for so long as possible and following intercurrent infections the child should be mobilised as early as possible since prolonged bedrest may lead to deterioration. One approach that has been found helpful is to try and prolong the period of ambulation by providing leg braces and by carrying out tenotomy, should this be necessary, to overcome contractures before the braces can be fitted (Spencer and Vignos, 1962). Once the child is chair-bound it is important that the back is maintained in a vertical position with a slightly backward incline to prevent the development of scoliosis. Supportive boots may assist in keeping the feet at a right angle and regular passive movements should be carried out to move the joints of the limbs through the full range of movement. In general physical activity is beneficial but exhaustion should be avoided and inactivity is generally detrimental. Obesity readily develops and considerably aggravates the disability; this should be prevented and treated if it arises by rigorous dieting. Once the patient is confined to a wheelchair it is important to provide appropriate aids such as a hydraulic lift if necessary, and where immobility is marked electronic aids such as the possum apparatus may be of particular value. Respiratory infection is a major cause of mortality and it is important to treat even apparently mild respiratory infections with appropriate antibiotics.

Genetic counselling

Duchenne dystrophy is inherited as an X-linked recessive. For this reason its occurrence is in males and it may be carried by clinically unaffected females. The carrier female will have a 50 per cent risk that any son she has is affected, and likewise there is a 50 per cent risk that any daughter may be a carrier. If a female is known to be a carrier appropriate genetic counselling can be provided. Should she become pregnant it is possible to determine the sex of the fetus at about 14 weeks gestation but it is not at present possible to determine whether a male fetus is affected by dystrophy or not. Furthermore, if the mother should elect to have a female child it must be borne in mind that any female child would have a 50 per cent chance of being a carrier.

If a female has an affected brother as well as an affected son she must be a definite carrier, and she is a probable carrier if she has an affected son but no siblings who are either clinically affected or carriers. Where possible carriers are concerned it is more difficult to determine the risk in precise terms. Thus the daughter of a definite carrier has a 50 per cent chance of being a carrier, but with the daughter of a possible carrier the risk is less and the risk may seem correspondingly less in the case of a female in a large family where there is only a single case. In these instances much help may be obtained from careful examination not only of the patient at risk but of as many close relatives as possible, since mild muscular weakness is not infrequently found in apparently healthy carriers. Likewise abnormality may be found by electromyography or in a muscle biopsy. The most useful single factor, however, is the detection of an elevated serum CPK since about 70 per cent of definite carriers have an elevated creatine phosphokinase. Where the CPK is markedly raised there can be very little doubt that the patient is a carrier; where, however, it is normal or very slightly elevated the situation may remain in doubt. Since so much depends on the finding it is essential to have several separate estimations of the creatine kinase in an individual patient. The estimations must be carried out by a reliable method and compared with a satisfactory set of control normal values. Blood should be taken off when the patient is at rest since high levels may be obtained after exercise. If the patient is pregnant it should be remembered that false low levels may be obtained. On the other hand high levels may be recorded in the newborn and higher than normal levels in young children.

Becker muscular dystrophy

In this less severe form of X-linked muscular dystrophy the general principles of management are similar to those of Duchenne dystrophy, bearing in mind that the disease may not present until the patient is in his teens or twenties and ambulation may continue well on into adult life. The same principles also apply to carrier detection but it is not certain at present how many carriers can be recognised by estimation of the serum creatine kinase.

Limb-girdle muscular dystrophy

The clinical course of limb-girdle muscular dystrophy is very variable but is frequently similar to that of the Becker type. Since many patients originally thought to have limb-girdle dystrophy have been found on careful study to have a different disorder such as spinal muscular atrophy, or a congenital myopathy or polymyositis, thorough investigation may be necessary to establish the diagnosis. The same general principles of management apply as to other forms of muscular dystrophy. Since the condition is generally transmitted as an autosomal recessive, both parents of an affected child must be heterozygotes so there is a 25 per cent chance that any further child may be affected. On the other hand the risk of a patient passing on the condition is very small as he or she is unlikely to marry a carrier unless he marries someone who is closely related. Occasionally limb-girdle dystrophy is inherited as an autosomal dominant and with any patient it is therefore important if possible to examine both parents to establish that neither parent is clinically affected.

Facioscapulohumeral muscular dystrophy

This is the most mild of the common varieties of muscular dystrophy and very little in the nature of physical treatment is generally required. Since the mobility of the scapula is one factor that impedes the use of the arms, sometimes orthopaedic measures to fixate the scapula may be of value. The condition is inherited as an autosomal dominant so that 50 per cent of the children of an affected parent are liable to be affected. In this condition some patients are so mildly affected that the condition is only recognised by careful clinical examination and careful examination is therefore necessary to establish whether a relative may not be a subclinically affected hererozygote.

Congenital muscular dystrophy

In this condition there is generally hypotonia and contractures are frequently present at birth but in others may develop subsequently. The condition is probably inherited as an autosomal recessive and may be only slowly progressive. Treatment should be directed to the correction of contractures. Passive stretching, the use of plaster calf casts and night splints and appropriate orthopaedic measures to achieve ambulation are important and every effort must be made to encourage full mobility.

MYOTONIA

The two most important conditions in which myotonia occurs are *myotonia congenita* (Thomsen's disease) and *dystrophia congenitica*. In both conditions inheritance is as an autosomal dominant but Becker has described a number of cases of myotonia congenita in which inheritance has been as an autosomal recessive (Harper and Johnston, 1972). In myotonia congenita there is little disability apart from the myotonia which has a tendency to improve as the patient grows older. Remedies which are effective in relieving myotonia include quinine, procainamide, phenytoin and corticosteroids, but all these medications carry side-effects and it can be questioned how far their use is justified as continued therapy unless the myotonia is of disabling severity. If any drug is necessary phenytoin is probably the drug of choice.

In *dystrophia myotonica* muscle weakness is a much more serious problem than the myotonia which seldom requires treatment. Inheritance is always as an autosomal dominant with very variable expression so that recognition of heterozygotes may be difficult. Transmission is through the mother or the father with approximately equal frequency but the infantile form is almost invariably transmitted through the mother, paternal transmission being commoner in the adult form.

The infantile form differs markedly from the adult form, marked hypotonia and difficulty in respiration being frequently present at birth when tube feeding may be necessary on account of difficulty in swallowing. Myotonia may be absent in infancy and children that survive tend to show marked motor retardation but once the neonatal period is passed the prognosis for life is relatively favourable. Accurate diagnosis is important because of the genetic risk that 50 per cent of any siblings are likely to be similarly affected, but may be difficult because myotonia may be absent in the infant and the mother is frequently very mildly affected.

In the adult form, as in other varieties of muscular dystrophy, no form of treatment will at present arrest the slowly progressive weakness of muscle. Many affected patients, however, have such mild disability that without careful examination the disease may pass undetected throughout life. On the other hand even mildly affected individuals may have other associated abnormalities such as cataract or conduction defects in the heart. Sudden death may occur particularly following anaesthesia (Gillam *et al.*, 1964) but also as a result of apparently un-heralded heart attacks; for this reason careful electrocardiographic screening both of patients and their close relatives should be carried out with a view to detecting bundle defects.

In genetic counselling the recognition of minimally affected hetero-zygotes is clearly important. The clinical detection of signs such as very mild facial weakness or percussion myotonia may be revealing, but in some individuals the only detectable abnormalities may be myotonia recorded electromyographically or cataract on slit-lamp examination. With any affected parent there is a 50 per cent chance that any children will be affected. The presence of linkage between the genes for myo-tonic dystrophy and the genes controlling the secretion of ABH blood group substances and also Lutheran blood group antigens provides the possibility for the antenatal detection of an affected fetus in a number of instances (Renwick *et al.*, 1971). Thus in a family which has the appropriate secretor status as determined by salivary testing it may be possible by determining the secretor status of the fetus by amniocen-tesis to ascertain whether it is likely to be affected by myotonic dys-trophy. Only about one-fifth of families have the appropriate secretor status for accurate prediction, and if the family is suitable the predic-tion carries an error approaching 10 per cent due to recombination (Harper, 1979; Roses *et al.*, 1979).

THE CONGENITAL MYOPATHIES

This is a varied group of disorders in which muscular weakness is present at birth or early infancy, often associated with hypotonia and with a variable distribution and a non-progressive or only slowly pro-gressive course. Clinical differentiation is rarely possible and diagnosis depends on histological and histochemical studies. Important varieties which have been described include central core disease, nemaline myo-pathy, centronuclear (myotubular) myopathy and the mitochondrial myopathies. Genetic counselling is difficult as few of the varieties have shown a consistent genetic pattern. Some families have been described with a dominant inheritance but there have been many sporadic cases and in some instances the pattern of inheritance has been recessive.

REFERENCES

Chou, S M and Gutmann, L (1970) Picornavirus-like crystals in subacute polymyositis. *Neurology (Minneapolis)*, **20** (1), 205—213.

Dawkins, R L (1965) Experimental myositis associated with hypersensitivity to muscle. *Journal of Pathology and Bacteriology*, **90**, 619—625.

Dubowitz, V (1978) *Muscle Disorders in Childhood*. W B Saunders, Philadelphia.

Ellis, F R, Clarke, I M C, Appleyard, T N and Dinsdale, R C W (1974) Malignant hyperpyrexia induced by nitrous oxide and treated with dexamethasone. *British Medical Journal*, **4**, 270—271.

Ellis, F R and Halsall, P S (1980) Malignant hyperpyrexia. *British Journal of Hospital Medicine*, **24**, 318—327.

Fernandez, J and Van de Kamer, J H (1968) Hexose and protein tolerance tests in children with liver glycogenosis caused by a deficiency of the debranching enzyme system. *Paediatrics*, **41**, 935—944.

Gillam, P M S, Heaf, P J D, Kaufman, L and Lucas, B G B (1964) Respiration in dystrophia myotonica. *Thorax*, **19**, 112—120.

Griggs, R G, Engel, W K and Resnick, S S (1970) Acetazolamide treatment of periodic paralysis. Prevention of attacks and improvement of persistent weakness. *Annals of Internal Medicine*, **73**, 39—48.

Harper, P S (1979) *Myotonic Dystrophy*. Saunders, Philadelphia and London.

Harper, P S and Johnston, D M (1972) Recessively inherited myotonia congenita. *Journal of Medical Genetics*, **9**, 213—215.

Isaacs, H and Barlow, M B (1973) Malignant hyperpyrexia. *Journal of Neurology, Neurosurgery and Psychiatry*, **36**, 228—243.

King, J O and Denborough, M A (1973) Malignant hyperpyrexia in Australia and New Zealand. *Medical Journal of Australia*, **1**, 525—528.

McArdle, B (1974) Metabolic and endocrine myopathies. In: *Disorders of Voluntary Muscle*, 3rd edn, pp. 726—759. (Ed) J N Walton. Churchill Livingstone, Edinburgh.

Mastaglia, F L and Walton, J N (1971) An ultrastructural study of skeletal muscle in polymyositis. *Journal of the Neurological Sciences*, **12**, 473—504.

Meyers, K R, Gilden, D H, Rinaldi, C F and Hansen, J L (1972) Periodic muscle weakness, normobalaemia and tubular aggregates. *Neurology (Minneapolis)*, **22**, 269—279.

Moulds, R F W and Denborough, M A (1972) Procaine in malignant hyperpyrexia. *British Medical Journal*, **4**, 526—528.

Moulds, R F W and Denborough, M A (1974) Biochemical basis of malignant hyperpyrexia. *British Medical Journal*, **2**, 241—244.

Müller, R and Kugelberg, E (1959) Myopathy in Cushing's syndrome. *Journal of Neurology, Neurosurgery and Psychiatry*, **22**, 314—319.

Pearson, C M and Currie, S (1974) Polymyositis and related disorders. In: *Disorders of Voluntary Muscle*, 3rd edn, pp. 614—652. (Ed) J N Walton. Churchill Livingstone, Edinburgh.

Perkoff, G T, Silber, R, Tyler, F H, Cartwright, G E and Wintrobe, M M (1959) Studies in disorders of muscle. XII. Myopathy due to the administration of therapeutic amounts of 17-hydroxycortico steroids. *American Journal of Medicine*, **26**, 891–898.

Poskanzer, D C and Kerr, D N S (1961) A third type of periodic paralysis, with normobalaemia and favourable response to sodium chloride. *American Journal of Medicine*, **31**, 328–342.

Ramsay, I D (1966) Muscle dysfunction in hypothyroidism. *Lancet*, **2**, 931–934.

Relton, J E S, Steward, D J, Creighton, R E and Britt, B A (1972) Malignant hyperpyrexia: a therapeutic and investigative regime. *Canadian Anaesthetists' Society Journal*, **19**, 200.

Renwick, S H, Bundey, S E, Ferguson-Smith, M A and Izatt, M M (1971) Confirmation of linkage of the loci for myotonic dystrophy and ABH secretion. *Journal of Medical Genetics*, **8**, 407–416.

Roses, A D, Harper, P S and Bossen, E H (1979) Myotonic muscular dystrophy. In: *Handbook of Clinical Neurology*. (Eds) P J Vinken and G W Bruyn; vol. 40: *Diseases of Muscle*, Part I (Eds) P J Vinken and G W Bruyn in collaboration with S P Ringel. North-Holland Publishing Company, Amsterdam.

Spencer, G E and Vignos, P J (1962) Bracing for ambulation in childhood progressive muscular dystrophy. *Journal of Bone and Joint Surgery*, **44A**, 234–242.

Viskoper, R J, Wolf, E, Chaco, J, Katz, R and Chowers, I (1975) McArdle's syndrome: the reaction to a fat-rich diet. *American Journal of the Medical Sciences*, **269**, 217–221.

Walton, J N and Gardner-Medwin, D (1974) Progressive muscular dystrophy and the myotonic disorders. In: *Disorders of Voluntary Muscle*, pp. 517–560. (Ed) J N Walton. Churchill Livingstone, Edinburgh.

CHAPTER FIFTEEN

Cervical and Lumbar Spondylosis and Cord Compression

Disease of the vertebral column is a common cause of neurological disability. This can come about through encroachment and pressure on nerve roots, from pressure on the spinal cord and from damage to the blood vessels leading to ischaemic changes in the cord and nerve roots. Degenerative changes in the cervical spine (cervical spondylosis) are a common cause of both radiculopathy and myelopathy. In the lumbar region arthritic changes and disc degeneration and protrusion can affect the lumbar and sacral roots and give rise to pain and weakness in the lower limbs. Both root irritation and myelopathy can also result from the effects of direct trauma, from abscess formation and from pressure by tumours, primary or secondary.

CERVICAL RADICULOPATHY

The development of severe pain in a root distribution in the neck or upper limb is commonly due to sudden protrusion of a soft piece of intervertebral cartilage and is effectively treated by rest in bed with immobilisation of the head between sandbags and using mild analgesics such as paracetamol or aspirin. If the pain continues in spite of rest, neck traction may be considered. Persistence of severe pain notwithstanding 2 weeks of neck traction may be an indication that surgical treatment is necessary. These acute disc protrusions may occur in healthy adults without radiological evidence of cervical spondylosis but following an abnormal or unusually sudden movement of the neck.

Less severe pain in a radicular distribution occurs fairly commonly in patients with cervical spondylosis. Here it is important to establish a precise diagnosis as root irritation may be the earliest symptom of a tumour presenting in relation to the cervical spine; likewise pain and paraesthesiae presenting in the upper limb may be due to an entrapment neuropathy affecting a peripheral nerve such as the median nerve in the carpal tunnel. Many mild cases of root irritation due to cervical spondylosis subside spontaneously without treatment but measures that may be effective include active shoulder girdle exercises, aimed to elevate the shoulder girdle and thus relieve tension on nerve roots and also to improve posture and strengthen the shoulder girdle muscles, and immobilisation of the neck in a plastic cervical collar. Many different types of collar are available and often acute symptoms can be effectively relieved by a temporary collar made of felt or plastic foam. The aim is to maintain the neck in a position of slight flexion with the chin indrawn, and commercially manufactured collars should be fitted carefully to make sure that the optimum position is maintained. Mild analgesics are useful and other forms of medical treatment include traction and manipulation. Traction may give immediate relief from pain when it is applied but often the pain recurs when the traction is relaxed. Neither traction nor manipulation are wholly free of hazard in patients with cervical spondylosis and different views have been summarised by Storey (1971). Relief from local muscle spasm may sometimes be achieved by local injection of hydrocortisone or local anaesthetic and by heat in the form of radiant heat or short-wave diathermy.

Referred pain from the cervical spine is often associated with a stiff (frozen) shoulder in which passive movement of the shoulder is painful and which may be associated with inflammation of the capsule of the joint. This condition is not entirely due to immobilisation because it may also occur in the presence of referred pain from other situations such as a myocardial infarct. It may also be associated with changes in the hand, which swells and becomes hot and painful with redness of the skin and later atrophy of the hand (Sudek's atrophy). The nature of this 'shoulder–hand syndrome' is not fully understood but it would seem likely that it includes some disturbance of the sympathetic system (Doret and Ferrero, 1951). In some cases an associated herpes zoster may be a factor but there seems little doubt that there is a strong correlation between the development of a frozen shoulder and dystrophic changes in the hand and cervical spondylosis. In treatment of cervical spondylosis it is therefore particularly important to maintain active mobilisation of the shoulder. When the stiffness has already developed active exercises sometimes supplemented by local injections of hydrocortisone should be carried out. Other measures which have been tried but are seldom indicated include stellate ganglion block and a course of therapy with oral prednisolone (Coventry, 1953; Graudal, 1959; Richardson, 1954; Steinbrocker *et al.*, 1953; Storey, 1971).

CERVICAL MYELOPATHY

Cervical myelopathy may develop in cervical spondylosis as a result of a variety of mechanisms. One is that degeneration of the intervertebral discs leads to shortening of the cervical spine with buckling of the posteriorly situated ligamentum flavum which can cause pressure on the cervical cord during flexion or extension of the spine. The cord may likewise be encroached on by a protruded intervertebral disc and these changes are particularly liable to give rise to problems in patients who already have a narrow cervical canal. Other factors include ischaemic changes in the cord as the result of constriction or damage to the blood vessels as they pass through the cervical spine. The myelopathy of cervical spondylosis generally presents as a slowly progressive spastic weakness involving first the lower limbs and then the arms. However other conditions can present in a similar way and the presence of radiological evidence of cervical spondylosis is not in itself sufficient to confirm the diagnosis since degenerative changes in the cervical spine without accompanying neurological disturbance are a frequent finding in adults over the age of 50. Multiple sclerosis may present in this way and when it does in an older person it is frequently accompanied by degenerative changes in the cervical spine but more often there are sphincter disturbances in the early stages. Examination of the cerebrospinal fluid with the finding of an elevated cell count or a raised γ-globulin and the demonstration of delayed visual evoked responses may be helpful in establishing this diagnosis. A tumour in relation to the cervical spine must also be considered and myelography may be necessary to rule this out.

Once the diagnosis of myelopathy due to cervical spondylosis is established it is useful to assess the response to medical treatment before considering the question of surgery. Sometimes a course of complete bed rest, with the patient lying flat on a hard bed with a low pillow for a period of 2–3 weeks, may bring symptomatic relief. In any patient, however, where the condition is clearly progressive surgical treatment must be considered. Investigation of a patient for surgery includes careful X-ray studies with measurements of the cervical canal and myelography. Symon (1971) has emphasised the importance of narrowing of the cervical canal in the recognition of cervical myelopathy severe enough to merit surgery. If the distance from the centre of the posterior wall of the vertebral body to the base of the spine of the same vertebra is measured patients with cervical myelopathy due to cervical spondylosis will frequently show a measurement at the narrowest point of the spine of 12 mm or less (Symon and Lavender, 1967).

Myelography may also show filling defects due to a disc protrusion or osteophytes or buckling of the ligamentum flavum. Changes of this nature in association with progressive clinical deterioration are an indication for surgical treatment as also may be exaggerated subluxation movement during flexion and extension of the neck.

Operative measures for the treatment of cervical spondylosis include foraminotomy for root pressure syndromes; and laminectomy for myelopathy, particularly where the cervical lordosis is exaggerated and there are multiple levels of spondylotic narrowing present and where limitation of movement is such that there is no significant instability of the spine and where the spinal canal is narrow. When the condition is localised to one or two intervertebral spaces, and when there is no marked narrowing of the rest of the spinal canal, an anterior fusion operation (Cloward, 1963) can be carried out. Assessment of the results of surgery is difficult because not all patients with cervical spondylotic myelopathy show a continuously progressive course in the absence of treatment and spontaneous remissions are not infrequent. Symon (1971) has reviewed the results in different published series and substantial numbers of cases have now been reported in which clinical improvement following operation included significant and rapid progress from a more severe to a lesser grade of disability.

LUMBAR SPONDYLOSIS

In the lumbar spine degenerative changes tend to be less marked than in the cervical spine but traumatic lesions occur quite frequently, particularly in young and active individuals leading to disc protrusion which is commonly lateral, affecting a single root but may also be central giving rise to pressure on the cauda equina. The commonest sites of lumbar disc protrusion are at L5,S1 and less frequently at L4,5 and usually L5 or S1 nerve roots are affected. The acute syndrome of a lateral disc protrusion includes back pain at the site and root pain usually in the distribution of the sciatic nerve. Generally the condition recovers spontaneously and the appropriate treatment is complete bed rest on a hard bed with a single pillow. If pain is severe continuous skin traction applied to the legs may give relief. As the condition improves the patient may be mobilised with back extension exercises and in severe cases a spinal support may prevent excessive movement once the patient resumes full activity. Surgical treatment may be indicated if an acute attack does not respond to rest and if continued pain is accompanied by progressive motor weakness, for example, in the dorsiflexors of the ankle. Recurrent episodes of sciatica may also be an indication for surgery. If a central disc protrusion is suspected with weakness of both lower limbs, absent ankle jerks and sphincter disturbance myelography is urgently indicated followed by surgical treatment, since paraplegia from a cauda equina lesion, once it has developed, may recover slowly if at all.

SPINAL CORD COMPRESSION

Spinal cord compression can develop gradually or acutely as a result of a disc protrusion, an abscess or a spinal tumour. About 20 per cent of spinal tumours are extradural and these are frequently malignant tumours of metastatic origin. The majority of spinal tumours are intradural and of these about 75 per cent are extramedullary; common extramedullary tumours are neurofibroma, meningioma or epidermoid. Intramedullary tumours include gliomata and vascular malformations. Acute cord compression is most commonly the result of a malignant extradural tumour although it can be due to an acute disc prolapse or to an extradural abscess. Slowly developing compression of the cord is more commonly the result of an intradural tumour which is frequently a benign surgically remediable lesion. Cord compression, however, from whatever cause — with the possible exception of a case of an elderly patient dying of cancer — is always an indication for surgical treatment. With acute cord compression investigation including myelography is of the greatest urgency, since if laminectomy is carried out before paraplegia is complete there is a good prospect that reasonable function may be preserved with relief of pain, even in the case of malignant extradural tumours. Following the removal of a benign extramedullary tumour the rate of recovery is very variable and sometimes it may be complete almost immediately; but many patients recover slowly and require active physiotherapy and measures of rehabilitation over an extended period of months.

An extradural spinal abscess most commonly occurs at the thoracolumbar junction and is usually due to a staphylococcal infection arising in the skin. In addition to rapidly developing paraplegia there may be backache associated with spinal tenderness and generally signs of infection such as a raised white blood cell count and ESR. In addition to urgent laminectomy and drainage of the pus high doses of systemic antibiotics must be given. The appropriate antibiotic will depend on bacterial sensitivity and before this is known an antibiotic effective against staphylococci should be employed.

SPINAL INJURY

The majority of spinal injuries are unaccompanied by neurological damage. Fracture dislocations of the spine particularly in the cervical region or thoracolumbar region can give rise to damage both to the spinal cord and to the roots, and it is important to distinguish between the two as root lesions may recover slowly by regeneration whereas severe spinal cord lesions once established can be expected to recover little or not at all. If the cord is mainly concussed recovery may be evident within the first 24 h and some function can be expected to have returned by 48 h. If the lesion is initially incomplete but shows progression then myelography and possibly surgical exploration is indicated.

Treatment of the patient with an established spinal cord injury is essentially the care of the paraplegic patient. In the early stages this requires the most meticulous medical and nursing management with a view to the prevention of complications while recovery from the spine injury takes place, and later progressive and active rehabilitation so that the patient can learn to live as normal a life as possible notwithstanding the disability (*see also* Chapter 7).

Care of the skin is essential to prevent the development of pressure sores. Because the paraplegic patient has lost skin sensation automatic movements to relieve the pressure of the skin no longer occur and careful positioning of the patient is necessary using special mattresses or foam-rubber pillows and taking great care to protect areas particularly prone to pressure such as the elbows, the lateral aspect of the hips, the heels and the skin over the scapulae. The patient should be turned every 2 h and the vulnerable areas should be washed and massaged. With an acute spinal injury, however, very great care must be taken in turning the patient if a fracture is thought to be present, particularly in the region of the cervical spine. A collar may prevent sudden movements of the neck, in particular flexion or extension, and if the patient is turned firm traction must be applied manually. With flexion injuries of the cervical spine continuous skull traction is advisable by means of skull calipers but with hyperextension injuries a collar will generally suffice.

The paraplegic patient generally develops retention of urine necessitating catheterisation. Alternative techniques are intermittent catheterisation with a strictly sterile technique or the use of an indwelling catheter. If the catheter is allowed to drain intermittently by releasing the clamp every 4 h the bladder is allowed to distend regularly and in some patients an automatic bladder may develop so that the bladder automatically empties itself every few hours whenever the internal pressure becomes adequate to excite the bladder reflex. In cases where an automatic bladder is not established, and generally this will be the case with lower motor neurone lesions which involve the sacral segments, some form of continuous drainage may be necessary. In some cases it is appropriate to exteriorise the ureters through an ileal loop and sometimes the patient may be taught self-catheterisation (*see* Chapter 7). In all cases active measures must be taken to control infection. If a catheter is in place daily washouts of the bladder with 1 in 5000 chlorhexidine may be helpful, and if infection develops the urine should be cultured and appropriate urinary antiseptics employed.

Retention of faeces usually occurs in paraplegic patients and initially enemas may be required every few days. Frequently, however, some degree of voluntary control over defaecation recovers and many patients can learn to provoke regular defaecation by means of a suppository.

Physiotherapy is vital both in respect of care of the limbs and care of the chest. The paralysed limbs must be put through the full range of movements every day and active physiotherapy is necessary to prevent contractures. Sometimes splints are necessary to prevent the development of deformities and flexor spasms may be treated by drugs such as diazepam 5–10 mg four times a day or baclofen initially 5 mg once a day increasing in divided doses up to 60–80 mg per day. Proper positioning of the limbs may be all-important in preventing the development of contractures and it is generally advisable to have a cage over the lower part of the bed to take the weight of the bedclothes. If spasticity is very severe so that contractures ultimately develop the position may be alleviated by judicious tenotomy or peripheral neurectomy, and in patients with complete spinal cord lesions intrathecal injections of phenol or alcohol may occasionally be indicated.

For a full discussion on spinal injuries the reader is referred to Guttman (1976).

REFERENCES

Cloward, R B (1963) Lesions of the intervertebral disc and their treatment by interbody fusion methods. The painful disc. *Clinical Orthopaedics*, **27**, 51–77.

Coventry, M B (1953) Problem of painful shoulder. *Journal of the American Medical Association*, **151**, 177–185.

Doret, J P and Ferrero, C (1951) Inegalité de la température cutanée dans l'infarctus du myocarde et l'angine de poitrine. *Cardiologia*, **19**, 80–96.

Guttman, L (1976) *Spinal cord injuries, comprehensive management and research*. Blackwell, Oxford.

Graudal, H (1959) Shoulder—hand syndrome and herpes zoster; report of a case with signs of vasodilatation and vasoconstriction in the same hand. *Acta Rheumatica Scandinavica*, 5, 157—163.

Richardson, A T (1954) Shoulder—hand syndrome following herpes zoster. *Annals of Physical Medicine*, 2, 132—134.

Steinbrocker, O, Neustadt, D H and Lapin, L (1953) Shoulder—hand syndrome — sympathetic block compared with corticotrophin and cortisone therapy. *Journal of the American Medical Association*, 153, 788—791.

Storey, G O (1971) Medical treatment. In: *Cervical Spondylosis*, pp. 140—153. (Ed) M Wilkinson. Heinemann, London.

Symon, L (1971) Surgical treatment. In: *Cervical Spondylosis*, 2nd edn, pp. 154—171. (Ed) M Wilkinson. Heinemann, London.

Symon, L and Lavender, P (1967) The surgical treatment of cervical myelopathy. *Neurology*, 17, 117—127.

Appendix—Adverse effects of drugs

PERIPHERAL NEUROPATHY

Antimicrobial
    chloramphenicol
    chloroquine
    clioquinol (withdrawn)
    colistin
    dapsone
    ethambutol
    ethionamide
    isoniazid
    metronidazole
    nitrofurantoin
    streptomycin
    sulphonamides

Antimitotic
    nitrogen mustards
    vincristine and vinblastine

Others
    arsenicals
    calcium carbimide
    disopyramide
    disulfiram
    emetine
    glutethimide
    gold
    hydrallazine
    imipramine

indomethacin
iproniazid (monoamine oxidase inhibitors)
methaqualone
perhexiline (demyelination)
phenytoin
thalidomide

OPTIC NEUROPATHY

chloramphenicol
chloroquine
ethambutol
isoniazid
sulphonamide
quinine
streptomycin (VIIIth nerve damage more common)

MYOPATHIC AND MYASTHENIC SYNDROMES

Subacute/chronic painless myopathy
    chloroquine (with neuropathy)
    heroin, alcohol (with neuropathy)
    steroids, especially fluorinated, e.g. triamcinolone

Hypokalaemia
    amphotericin B
    carbenoxolone
    diuretics
    purgatives

Acute or subacute painful myopathy
    alcohol
    amphetamine
    cimetidine
    clofibrate
    emetine
    epsilon-aminocaproic acid
    heroin

isoetharine
vincristine (with neuropathy)

Acute rhabdomyolysis
alcohol
amphetamine
heroin
phencyclidine

Syndrome of cramps, myalgia and/or weakness
bumetanide
clofibrate
cytotoxic drugs
isoetharine
lithium
salbutamol

Polymyositis or dermatomyositis
penicillamine

Myotonic syndrome
propranolol
suxamethonium

Myasthenic syndromes (production or precipitation)
aminoglycosides (gentamycin, streptomycin, etc.)
chlorpromazine
penicillamine
phenytoin
polymyxins
procainamide
propranolol
trimethadione

BENIGN INTRACRANIAL HYPERTENSION

nalidixic acid
oral contraceptives
steroids

tetracyclines
vitamin A intoxication

CONVULSIONS (PRECIPITATION OR EXACERBATION)

cephalosporins
cycloserine
disopyramide
haloperidol
hypoglycaemic agents: e.g. chlorpropamide
isoniazid
lignocaine
lithium
monoamine oxidase inhibitors
nalidixic acid
penicillins
phenothiazines
tricyclic antidepressants

TOXIC CONFUSIONAL STATE

anticholinergics
barbiturates
benzodiazepines
carbamazepine
lignocaine
lithium
methyl dopa
monoamine oxidase inhibitors
narcotic analgesics
phenothiazines
phenytoin
tricyclic antidepressants

MOVEMENT DISORDERS

Akathisia (motor restlessness)
  butyrophenones
  L-dopa

phenothiazines
thiothixenes

Choreoathetosis
L-dopa
lithium
phenothiazines
phenytoin

Dystonia
butyrophenones
L-dopa
metoclopramide
phenothiazines

Parkinsonism
butyrophenones
lithium
phenothiazines
reserpine
tetrabenazine

Tardive dyskinesia
phenothiazines
butyrophenones

Tremor
alcohol
amphetamine
lithium
methylphenidate
monoamine oxidase inhibitors
sodium valproate
tricyclic drugs

Cerebellar syndrome
barbiturates
carbamazepine
5-fluorouracil
lithium
phenytoin

Index